Running Mechanics and Gait Analysis

Reed Ferber, PhD, CAT(C), ATC

Running Injury Clinic, University of Calgary, Alberta

Shari Macdonald, MSc, BScPT

Running Injury Clinic, Calgary, Alberta

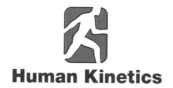

Human Kinetics

Library of Congress Cataloging-in-Publication Data

Ferber, Reed, 1970- author.
  Running mechanics and gait analysis / Reed Ferber, Shari Lynn Macdonald.
    p. ; cm.
  Includes bibliographical references and index.
  I. Macdonald, Shari Lynn, 1970- author. II. Title.
  [DNLM: 1. Running--physiology. 2. Athletic Injuries--prevention & control. 3. Gait--physiology.
QT 260.5.R9]
  QP310.R85
  612'.044--dc23

2013035718

ISBN-13: 978-1-4504-2439-4 (print)

The web addresses cited in this text were current as of October 24, 2013, unless otherwise noted.

Acquisitions Editors: Melinda Flegel and Joshua J. Stone; **Developmental Editor:** Katherine Maurer; **Assistant Editor:** Susan Huls; **Copyeditor:** Claire Marty; **Indexer:** Laurel Plotzke; **Permissions Manager:** Dalene Reeder; **Graphic Designer:** Joe Buck; **Graphic Artist:** Kathleen Boudreau-Fuoss; **Cover Designer:** Keith Blomberg; **Photograph (cover):** © Human Kinetics; **Photographs (interior):** courtesy of the authors unless otherwise noted; **Photo Asset Manager:** Laura Fitch; **Visual Production Assistant:** Joyce Brumfield; **Photo Production Manager:** Jason Allen; **Art Manager:** Kelly Hendren; **Associate Art Manager:** Alan L. Wilborn; **Illustrations:** © Human Kinetics; **Printer:** McNaughton & Gunn

Printed in the United States of America   10 9 8 7 6 5

The paper in this book is certified under a sustainable forestry program.

Human Kinetics
1607 N. Market Street
Champaign, IL 61820
USA

United States and International
Website: **US.HumanKinetics.com**
Email: info@hkusa.com
Phone: 1-800-747-4457

Canada
Website: **Canada.HumanKinetics.com**
Email: info@hkcanada.com

E5660

Tell us what you think!
Human Kinetics would love to hear what we can do to improve the customer experience. Use this QR code to take our brief survey.

Contents

Preface   v
Accessing the Online Video   ix
Acknowledgments   xi

Chapter 1   Incidence of Running-Related Injuries   1

Defining an Overuse Injury. 2
Etiology of Overuse Injuries in Runners 2
Common Running-Related Injuries 4
Understanding Clinical and Biomechanical Risk Factors 7
Summary 8

Chapter 2   Assessing Foot Mechanics   9

Biomechanics 10
Atypical Foot Mechanics and Injury .15
Strength 16
Anatomical Alignment. 18
Flexibility 20
Summary 22

Chapter 3   Footwear Selection   23

Overview of Running Shoes. 24
Footwear Research Findings 26
Shoe Fitting 28
Barefoot Running. 31
Orthotic Devices and Foot Mechanics 33
Summary 35

Chapter 4   Assessing Knee Mechanics   37

Biomechanics 38
Strength 41
Anatomical Alignment. 44
Flexibility 47
Summary 48

Chapter 5   Assessing Hip Mechanics   49

Biomechanics 50
Strength 52
Anatomical Alignment 54
Flexibility 56
Summary 61

**Chapter 6   Proximal to Distal Relationships:
Case Studies   63**

Torsional Forces 64
Frontal Plane Mechanics 72
Summary 84

Chapter 7   Can We Influence Gait Mechanics?   85

Feedback 86
Strength Training 88
Revisiting the Case Studies 88
Summary 89

**Chapter 8   Overview of Clinical and Biomechanical
Assessment   91**

Foot, Ankle, and Tibia 92
Knee 94
Hip 96
Summary 98

Chapter 9   Technical Aspects of Video Gait Analysis   99

Sampling Frequency 100
F-Stop and Shutter Speed 102
Software Options 103
Summary 103

Afterword   105
Appendix: Terminology for Gait Biomechanics   107
Glossary   111
References   117
Index   131
About the Authors   139

Preface

Running continues to be the most popular physical activity in North America with over 50 million estimated participants. However, various epidemiological studies have estimated that anywhere from 27% to 70% of recreational and competitive distance runners sustain an overuse running injury during any one-year period. With an estimated 16% of North Americans participating in a recreational running program (Institute 2009), approximately 27 million adults will experience a running-related injury each year, resulting in over $35 billion in direct costs (Knowles 2007). Thus, health care professionals, coaches, and runners should be educated on the multifactorial nature of running injuries for the purpose of injury prevention and optimal treatment.

The knee is the most common site of injury, representing 40% of all running-related injuries, and patellofemoral pain syndrome (PFPS) accounts for 46% to 62% of those injuries. Since 35% of North Americans participate in running-related activities, 48 to 62 million adults will be affected by a PFPS injury in any given year. Thus, the ability to understand the underlying factors that contribute to injuries such as PFPS is critical for prevention and developing optimal rehabilitation protocols.

For an injured runner, several options are available for treatment. In many cases, clinicians perform some form of gait analysis to better understand how the patient's underlying walking and running mechanics are related to etiology of injury. However, the multifactorial nature of any running injury demands that the clinician be well trained and understand the interrelationships between gait biomechanics, anatomical alignment, muscular strength, and muscular flexibility. Looking at any one of these factors in isolation does not adequately provide clinicians with the answers needed for optimizing the rehabilitation protocol for the patient or the information necessary for preventing injury recurrence. Therefore, this book provides an overview of the most recent research and clinical concepts related to gait and injury analysis.

We have written this book primarily for physical therapists and athletic trainers who are involved in the clinical assessment and treatment of running-related injuries. However, personal trainers and coaches will also significantly benefit from this book, since many of the concepts are related to preventing injuries and improving running performance. Finally, average runners will also glean a tremendous amount of knowledge from this book so long as they have some knowledge of biomechanics and a passion for learning.

In chapter 1, we provide an overview of the epidemiology research and discuss the fact that despite significant advances in running shoe technology, training programs, and research, running injuries have not decreased over the past 35 years. In fact, some injuries, such as iliotibial band syndrome and stress fractures, have doubled in that time. We discuss common signs and symptoms associated with the most common running-related injuries and present the relevant research to help you distinguish and identify these common injuries. Moreover, we introduce the concept that four factors must be considered in order to understand the root cause of an injury: measures of gait biomechanics, muscular strength, tissue flexibility, and anatomical alignment.

The subsequent chapters provide in-depth analysis of typical and atypical foot, knee, hip, and pelvis running biomechanics. With the confusion and mis-interpretation about basic foot biomechanics, we start in chapter 2 with basic definitions of foot pronation and supination and an understanding of overall foot mechanics. A discussion about current literature related to footwear prescrip-tion, categories of running shoes, how running shoes influence foot mechanics, and minimalist shoes and barefoot running are covered in chapter 3. Moving up the kinematic chain, knee and hip biomechanics are discussed with respect to foot mechanics in chapters 4 and 5. Specific research related to how atypical foot mechanics influence knee and hip injuries is discussed along with novel approaches to understanding and identifying atypical joint forces. In keeping with the four factors that must be considered for any injury assessment, we present how anatomical alignment, muscle strength, and tissue flexibility are all interrelated and influence ankle, foot, knee, and hip biomechanics.

Once the complexities of gait biomechanics are systematically discussed and dissected and methods for injury assessment are outlined, we provide three case studies in chapter 6, including scientific summaries of each patient's running biomechanics along with the measures of strength, flexibility, and anatomical alignment so that you can gain some real-world experience in injury assess-ment. Proximal to distal relationships of torsional (twisting) and frontal plane (collapsing) forces and how they relate to common running-related injuries are discussed in depth.

Moving toward the rehabilitation aspects of running injuries, in chapter 7 the question of whether we can influence gait mechanics is answered in the context of novel treatment techniques that have been developed, including real-time feedback. In contrast to these novel technologies, we investigate recent research to see if muscle strengthening exercises can also cause alterations in lower-extremity biomechanics and thus optimize injury treatment.

In chapter 8, we summarize information covered in earlier chapters in tables that display the relationships of the kinetic chain interactions and structural, strength, and flexibility issues that accompany atypical movement patterns of the feet, knees, and legs. Finally, the ability to perform a gait analysis demands the proper equipment and knowledge about the technical aspects. In chapter 9, we discuss research and technical concepts so that you can purchase the correct video camera and use it effectively. We also provide an overview of commercially available software.

With this book, you have access to video clips of runners who exhibit both typical and atypical joint motions. These clips make the connection from text to practice and improve your ability to identify movement patterns and analyze running gait.

Our goal is to provide a more thorough understanding of the complexities of running biomechanics and the interrelationships of muscular strength, flexibility, and anatomical alignment for the purpose of providing an advanced clinical assessment of gait. Most important, the underlying theories put forth are grounded in the most current biomechanical and clinical research to provide valuable and innovative tools to improve clinical practice and the ability to rehabilitate and prevent running injuries. We reference more than 250 peer-reviewed scientific manuscripts throughout the textbook and include the most up-to-date research. We know of no other resource that contains a comprehensive list of running-related research.

COMPREHENSIVE APPROACH DEVELOPED BY THE RUNNING INJURY CLINIC

For over 10 years our team of clinical scientists, mechanical and biomedical engineers, clinicians, and biomechanists have been researching and developing novel scientific assessment techniques for running and walking injuries. The purpose of our applied research laboratory is to improve our understanding of etiology of injury and optimal treatment. However, this book is not just a discussion of our approach. Rather, the techniques and rationale for the selected variables of interest discussed throughout this book are based on our research as well as research from other laboratories around the world. Based on this approach, it is not our opinion we are providing in this textbook. Rather, it is our scientific approach, the basis for our decision-making process, and the rationale for our judgment regarding the root cause of a musculoskeletal injury.

At the Running Injury Clinic, we measure selected strength, flexibility, and anatomical alignment variables using scientific devices and combine these variables with 3-dimensional (3D) measures of walking and running gait. Considering that most clinicians do not have access to a 3D motion capture system, this book provides methods that relate the measurable biomechanical variables (i.e., rearfoot eversion) to the nonmeasurable (i.e., tibial internal rotation).

This book is a compilation of biomechanical research and research involving healthy and injured individuals. Since this is a new area of research, and very few studies have taken a comprehensive approach to understanding the interrelationship between clinical and biomechanical factors, we are limited in terms of resources to pull from. Regardless, the mechanics of walking and running are mostly similar aside from the flight phase of running and the subsequent increased impact sustained. As research continues to evolve, we will continue to update this book with the latest information from around the world.

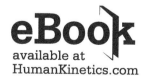

eBook
available at
HumanKinetics.com

Accessing the Online Video

This book includes access to online streaming video, including more than 30 video clips of runners illustrating 15 of the biomechanical patterns and case studies discussed in the text. Audio descriptions provided by the authors break down details of the runners' movements and will help you apply concepts from this text to real-life clinical scenarios. Throughout this text, special notes marked with a play button icon indicate where the content is supplemented by online video clips.

You can access the online video by visiting www.HumanKinetics.com/ RunningMechanicsAndGaitAnalysis. Click on the first edition link next to the book cover. Click the Sign In link on the left or top of the page. If you do not have an account with Human Kinetics, you will be prompted to create one.

If the online video does not appear in the Ancillary Items box on the left of the page, click the Enter Pass Code option in that box. Enter the pass code that is printed here, including all hyphens. Click the Submit button to unlock the online video. After you have entered this pass code the first time, you will never have to enter it again. For future visits, all you need to do is sign in to the book's website and follow the link that appears in the left menu!

Pass code for online video: FERBER-MHMLYJ-0SG

Once you have signed into the site and entered the pass code, select Online Video in the ancillary items box in the upper-left corner of the screen. You'll then see an Online Video page with information about the video. Select the link to open the online video web page. On the online video page, you will see a set of buttons that correspond to the chapters in the text that have accompanying video. Select the button for the chapter's videos you want to watch. Once you select a chapter, a player will appear. In the player, the clips for that chapter will appear vertically along the right side, numbered as they are in the text. Select the video you would like to watch and view it in the main player window. You can use the buttons at the bottom of the main player window to view the video full screen and to pause, fast-forward, or reverse the clip.

Following is a list of the clips included in the online video.

Video 2.1a-c Typical foot mechanics

Video 2.2 Excessive eversion

Video 2.3 Prolonged eversion

Video 2.4a-b Excessive eversion velocity

Video 2.5a-b Reduced foot mechanics

Video 4.1a-c Typical knee mechanics

Video 4.2a-d Excessive knee genu valgum (abduction)

Video 4.3 Excessive knee flexion

Video 4.4 Reduced knee flexion

Video 5.1a-b Typical hip mechanics

Video 5.2a-c Excessive hip adduction (pelvic drop)

Video 6.1 Medial heel whip

Video 6.2a-b Runner with tibialis posterior tendinopathy (case study)

Video 6.3a-e Runner with medial tibial stress syndrome (case study)

Video 6.4a-b Runner with patellofemoral pain syndrome (case study)

Acknowledgments

Dr. Ferber's research is primarily funded through his Population Health New Investigator Award from Alberta Innovates: Health Solutions (funded by the Alberta Heritage Foundation for Medical Research endowment fund). Other research awards also provide significant support for the lab and have come through the National Athletic Trainers' Association Research and Education Foundation, Alberta Innovates: Technology Futures, Worker's Compensation Board of Alberta, Olympic Oval High Performance Fund at the University of Calgary, and a very generous charitable donation from SOLE Inc.

We thank Dr. Kathryn Mills for providing editorial assistance and extend a heartfelt thank-you to all of the students and staff who work in the Running Injury Clinic at the University of Calgary. Thanks for your hard work and dedication to our research and clinical program.

Incidence of Running-Related Injuries

Although runners occasionally sustain acute injuries such as ankle sprains and muscle strains, the majority of running injuries can be classified as cumulative microtrauma (overuse) injuries. Running is one of the most popular activities, and overuse injuries of the lower extremity occur regularly. There is no agreed-on standardized definition of an overuse running injury, but several authors have defined it as a musculoskeletal ailment attributed to running that causes a restriction of running speed, distance, duration, or frequency for a least 1 week (Koplan et al. 1982; Macera et al. 1989; Hreljac et al. 2000). Using slight variations of this definition, various epidemiological studies have estimated that 27% to 70% of recreational and competitive distance runners sustain an overuse running injury during any 1-year period (Caspersen et al. 1984; Jacobs and Berson 1986; Lysholm and Wiklander 1987; Marti et al. 1988; Walter et al. 1989; Rochcongar et al. 1995). The runners in these studies vary considerably in their running experience and training habits, but generally they run a minimum distance of 20 km per week (12 mi per week) on a regular basis and have been running consistently for at least one to three years.

DEFINING AN OVERUSE INJURY

An overuse injury to the musculoskeletal system results from the combined fatigue effect over a period of time beyond the capabilities of the stressed structure (Stanish 1984; Elliott 1990). Although repeated stresses on various structures of the musculoskeletal system may result in an overuse injury, this does not imply that stresses to the musculoskeletal system should be minimized to avoid injury. All biological structures, such as muscles, tendons, ligaments, and bones, adapt both positively and negatively to the level of stress placed on them. Positive adaptation occurs when the applied stresses are repeated below the mechanical limits of a structure and adequate time periods are provided between stress applications (Kannus et al. 1994; Bailon-Plaza and van der Meulen 2003). On the other hand, negative adaptation (injury) occurs when a stress is applied beyond the mechanical limits either one time, as in the case of an acute injury, or repeated times with an insufficient time period between stress applications, as with overuse injuries (Stanish 1984; Elliott 1990; Rolf 1995).

ETIOLOGY OF OVERUSE INJURIES IN RUNNERS

The training variables most often identified as risk factors for overuse running injuries include running distance, training intensity, rapid increases in weekly running distance or intensity, and stretching habits (James, Bates et al. 1978; Jacobs and Berson 1986; Marti et al. 1988; Messier and Pittala 1988; Paty 1994; James 1998; Plastarasv et al. 2005). Examining how these variables affect the stress–frequency relationship reveals how some of these training variables may lead to overuse injuries (figure 1.1). Increasing running distance increases the number of repetitions of the applied stress since the number of steps taken increases. Provided that running speed remained unchanged, the magnitude

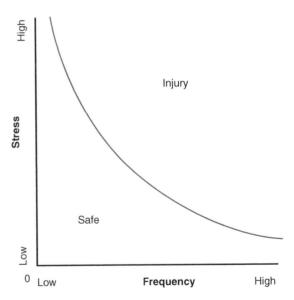

Figure 1.1 Overuse injury occurrence due to the theoretical relationship between stress application and frequency of force application.

of the forces and moments produced at various musculoskeletal structures during each step remain unchanged also (neglecting fatigue effects). Thus, running a greater distance places the involved musculoskeletal structures further to the right on the graph by increasing the number of stress applications. Since this portion of the curve has a slight negative slope, locations further to the right on the curve require slightly lower stresses for a structure to enter the injury zone of the curve. Thus, the possibility that one or more structures will enter the injury zone of the graph increases with increasing running distance.

In running, training intensity relates to running speed. Faster running speeds generally produce greater forces and torsional stress to the involved musculoskeletal structures (Hamill et al. 1982; Nigg 1986; Derrick et al. 2000; Mercer et al. 2002). When training intensity increases, the stress level applied to all of these structures occurs higher on the stress-frequency graph (figure 1.1). Locations higher on this graph require fewer repetitions for a structure to enter the injury zone. In this way, when training intensity increases without a decrease in running distance or frequency, the likelihood of injury also increases.

The stress–frequency relationship can also explain how rapid changes in distance or intensity increase the risk of injury. When a musculoskeletal structure is subjected to a stress-frequency combination that is close to the stress–frequency curve yet below or to the left of the curve, positive remodeling of the structure may occur, shifting the curve upward and to the right as long as detraining does not occur. When these increases in running distance and intensity are gradual, it is possible to shift the stress–frequency curve to outpace the shifting of the structure's location on the graph. However, rapid increases in running distance or intensity may cause the structure to cross the curve from the non-injury region to the injury region even when some positive remodeling and shifting of the curve has occurred.

Performing stretching exercises before running is a training-related variable that has been examined as a possible risk factor for running injuries. Unfortunately, there have been conflicting conclusions drawn regarding the association of this factor with overuse running injuries. A number of researchers have reported that people who stretch regularly before running experience a higher rate of injury than those who do not stretch regularly (Jacobs and Berson 1986; Hart et al. 1989; Rochcongar et al. 1995). On the other hand, others have not found an association between stretching before running and injuries (Blair et al.1987; Macera et al. 1989; Hreljac et al. 2000). No empirical studies have reported that regular stretching before running reduces the number of running injuries, even though this practice has been advocated as a means of preventing running injuries (van Mechelen et al. 1993). However, data related to the stretching and warm-up habits of runners generally rely on surveys or self-reporting, so these results must be considered cautiously. Indeed, it is very possible that stretching before running is important for some runners, while it may not be necessary for others. A systematic review and meta-analysis by Yeung and Yeung (2001) reported that research investigating protocols of stretching before exercise and stretching outside the training sessions did not produce a clinically useful or statistically significant reduction in the risk of soft tissue running-related injuries. Without conclusive evidence, other factors, such as training errors, should be considered first as potential contributors to injury.

Several clinical studies have estimated that over 60% of overuse running injuries are a result of variables related to training (Clement et al. 1981; Lysholm and Wiklander 1987; Kibler 1990; Macintyre et al. 1991). From a practical standpoint, it could be stated that *all* overuse running injuries are attributable to training variables. To sustain an overuse injury, a runner must have subjected some musculoskeletal structure to a stress–frequency combination that crossed over to the injury zone of the current stress–frequency curve for the injured structure. This can only be accomplished when an individual exceeds the current limit of running distance or intensity in such a way that the negative remodeling of the injured structure predominates over the repair process. The exact *location* of this limit would vary from structure to structure and from individual to individual, but there is no doubt that runners can prevent these injuries by training differently based on individual limitations or in some cases by not training at all.

One of the most appealing aspects of assigning the causes of all overuse running injuries to training variables is that all of these injuries could then be considered preventable, since runners have control over training variables. However, rarely do runners know that they are about to commit a training error that will place them outside of their injury threshold. Therefore, to prevent overuse running injuries and assess and understand the etiology of a current injury, knowledge of the current limits of all of the involved musculoskeletal structures is required. These limits primarily are determined by anatomical and biomechanical variables in addition to the current state of training, strength and flexibility of specific tissues and muscles, and the integrity and injury status of various structures. Of course, it is not possible to know these limits exactly, but it is possible to minimize the risk of injury by thoroughly understanding the key clinical and biomechanical risk factors.

This book provides clinicians with a thorough and scientifically grounded basis so that they can make evidence-based decisions about these clinical and biomechanical factors. With this in mind, we discuss the most common running injuries and their multifactorial nature based on the current research.

COMMON RUNNING-RELATED INJURIES

The knee is the most common site of overuse running injuries, accounting for close to half of all running injuries (Clement et al. 1981; Pinshaw et al. 1984; Rolf 1995; Taunton et al. 2002). According to a clinical study of more than 2,000 injured runners (Taunton et al. 2002), 42% had knee injuries, 92% had lower leg injuries, and 22% had injuries superior to the knee. The most common knee injury was patellofemoral pain syndrome and was seen in 331 individuals, followed by iliotibial band friction syndrome (168 cases), plantar fasciitis (158 cases), meniscal injuries (100 cases), and patellar tendinitis (96 cases) (see table 1.1). Other researchers have reported a fairly similar breakdown for the location of overuse running injuries (Clement et al. 1981; Marti et al. 1988; Rolf 1995). Although very few overuse running injuries have an established etiology (Rolf 1995), the fact that over 80% of these injuries occur at or below the knee suggests that there may be some common mechanisms.

In the next sections, we discuss the top two running-related injuries, patellofemoral pain syndrome and iliotibial band syndrome, as examples of the complexity of understanding the root cause of a running injury. Through this discussion, we outline the pathomechanics and interrelationships between strength, alignment, and flexibility.

Patellofemoral Pain Syndrome

Patellofemoral pain syndrome (PFPS) is one of the most common injuries in running and jumping sports regardless of age or sex. In a survey of patient chart data from cases of running and jumping-based sports that were referred to an outpatient sports medicine clinic over a 5-year period, PFPS was one of the most common injuries for adults aged 22 to 38 years (Matheson et al. 1989). Activities for these individuals included recreational running, fitness classes, field sports, and racket sports. With respect to running, the knee has been shown to be the most common site of injury, representing approximately 40% of all running-related injuries, and PFPS accounts for 46% to 62% of these injuries (Clement and Taunton 1981; Pinshaw et al. 1984; Taunton et al. 2002).

While PFPS is a common problem experienced by active adults (Brody and Thein 1998; Thomee et al. 1999), the etiology of PFPS has remained vague and controversial (Powers 1998; Dye et al. 1999; Witvrouw et al. 2000; Naslund et al.

Table 1.1 Frequency of the 10 Most Common Injuries in a Study of Injured Runners

Injury	Frequency of injury
Patellofemoral syndrome	16.5%
Iliotibial band syndrome	8.40%
Plantar fasciitis	7.80%
Tibial stress syndrome	4.94%
Patellar tendinitis	4.80%
Achilles tendinitis	4.80%
Gluteus medius injuries	3.50%
Tibial stress fracture	3.30%
Hamstring injuries	2.29%

Data from Taunton and Ryan 2002.

2005; Witvrouw et al. 2005). Unlike other knee dysfunctions such as an anterior cruciate ligament injury, which often have a specific onset and mechanism of injury, patients with PFPS generally report diffuse peripatellar and retropatellar pain of an insidious onset. In addition, the majority of patients often report pain with no discernable cause other than overuse (Dye et al. 1999; Dye 2001; Fulkerson 2002). Dye (2001) has described PFPS as an orthopedic enigma because of the continued misunderstanding of its etiology. Thus, a thorough understanding of all etiological factors is essential for properly treating and preventing this common injury.

For example, female runners are twice as likely to sustain PFPS compared to their male counterparts (Taunton et al. 2002; Ferber et al. 2003). One study reported that female runners exhibit increased hip internal rotation angle, which likely led to a reduced peak external **knee rotation** (rotation of the distal femur on the tibia) angle compared to men (Ferber et al. 2003). In addition, female runners remained in greater amounts of tibial external rotation compared to men throughout the entire stance phase of gait. These results are in support of Yoshioka et al. (1989) who reported that women exhibit greater static external knee rotation alignment compared to men. Moreover, Tiberio (1987) suggested that excessive internal rotation of the femur may result in malalignment of the patellofemoral joint and lead to anterior knee pain. The increased hip internal rotation demonstrated by the female runners in the aforementioned study by Ferber et al. 2003, coupled with the greater **knee abduction (genu valgum)** may result in a greater dynamic **Q-angle**. An increase in the Q-angle is thought to result in higher patellofemoral joint contact forces and place a runner at greater risk for injury (Cowan et al. 1996; Mizuno et al. 2001). These results, amongst others, may also partially explain why female runners are twice as likely to develop PFPS (DeHaven and Lintner 1986; Almeida et al. 1999). See chapter 4 for a more in-depth discussion of the influence of Q-angle.

Iliotibial Band Syndrome

Iliotibial band syndrome (ITBS) is the second leading cause of knee pain in runners and the most common cause of lateral knee pain (Noble 1980; Taunton et al. 2002). Anecdotally, this syndrome has been associated with repetitive flexion and extension on a loaded knee in combination with a tight iliotibial band (Noble 1980; Orchard et al. 1996; Birnbaum et al. 2004; Miller et al. 2007; Noehren et al. 2007). Orchard et al. (1996) suggested that frictional forces between the iliotibial band and the lateral femoral condyle are greatest at 20° to 30° of **knee flexion**, which occurs during the first half of the stance phase of running. However, despite this well-accepted sagittal plane theory (Noble 1980; Orchard et al. 1996; Birnbaum et al. 2004), no differences have been found in the few biomechanical investigations involving knee flexion and extension patterns in runners who had ITBS compared to healthy controls (Miller et al. 2007; Noehren et al. 2007; Ferber et al. 2010).

It is possible that motions in other planes or at other joints may contribute to ITBS. The primary functions of the iliotibial band are to serve as a lateral hip and knee stabilizer and to resist **hip adduction** and knee internal rotation (Fredericson et al. 2000; Moore and Dalley 2005). As a result of the femoral and tibial attachments, it is possible that abnormal hip as well as foot mechanics, which both influence the knee, could play a role in the development of ITBS. For example, a study reported that female recreational runners who had previously sustained ITBS exhibited significantly greater stance phase peak hip adduction and peak knee internal rotation angles compared with a control group during running (see figure 1.2) (Ferber et al. 2010). These results were similar to those reported for a prospective study conducted in the same laboratory environment with a separate group of subjects (Noehren et al. 2007). The common results between the prospective study and the retrospective study provide strong evidence related to atypical running mechanics and the etiology

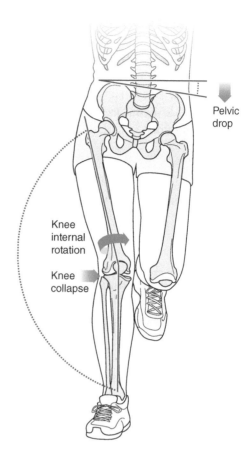

Figure 1.2 A runner exhibiting a combination of excessive pelvic drop, knee collapse, and knee rotation.

of ITBS. However, other factors, such as reduced hip abductor muscle strength (Fredericson et al. 2000; Ireland et al. 2003; Niemuth et al. 2005) and atypical anatomical alignment (Horton and Hall 1989), may also play a role in the development of this particular injury.

UNDERSTANDING CLINICAL AND BIOMECHANICAL RISK FACTORS

Although there has been a large amount of speculation regarding the mechanisms of running injuries, the exact causes of overuse running injuries have yet to be determined. It could only be stated with certainty that the etiology of these injuries is multifactorial and diverse (Marti et al. 1988; Rolf 1995; van Mechelen 1995). It has occasionally been suggested that particular running injuries, or sites of injuries, are associated with specific risk factors, but some researchers have concluded that there are no specific risk factors that correlate with specific types of injury in a reliable fashion (James and Jones 1990; James 1998). However, different research studies have investigated various risk factors in isolation and have provided reasonable rationale as to why they may be associated with a variety of running injuries.

To provide a comprehensive injury assessment for a running-related injury, four factors must be considered:

1. Biomechanical gait patterns
2. Muscular strength
3. Anatomical alignment
4. Tissue flexibility

Throughout this book, we discuss each of these four variables and provide a review of the scientific literature. For each variable we provide scientific data on typical and atypical limits or measures for each so that the clinician can replicate, to the best of their abilities and equipment available, an injury assessment similar to what we perform at the Running Injury Clinic at the University of Calgary.

SUMMARY

Now that we've defined a running injury, discussed some of the common running injuries runners sustain, and discussed etiology of injury, it's time to go more in depth into the pathomechanics and interrelationships between strength, alignment, and flexibility. Based on the brief discussion regarding ITBS and PFPS, running injuries are complex. Thus, we need to develop a systematic approach to clinical gait assessment and understanding these interrelationships. We start from the foot and work upward. Chapter 2 begins with an in-depth discussion of foot mechanics.

CHAPTER

2

Assessing Foot Mechanics

To develop a systematic method for clinical gait assessment, we discuss biomechanical, strength, anatomical, and flexibility factors based on the most up-to-date research literature. We begin with the foot because most research over the past 20 years has focused on mechanics of foot pronation and because the shock wave or ground reaction force begins at the foot as it moves up the kinematic chain.

BIOMECHANICS

The stance phase of walking or running gait can be divided into two functional phases. The first half of stance is commonly referred to as the cushioning, or eccentric, phase of gait. The last half of stance is referred to as the propulsion, or concentric phase. When the foot strikes the ground, it is supinated, or locked, to better attenuate the initial shock wave traveling up into the foot. Just before midstance the foot pronates, or unlocks. Then, as the heel lifts off the ground in preparation for toe-off, the foot once again supinates to allow the first ray to become a rigid lever to propel the runner forward (figure 2.1).

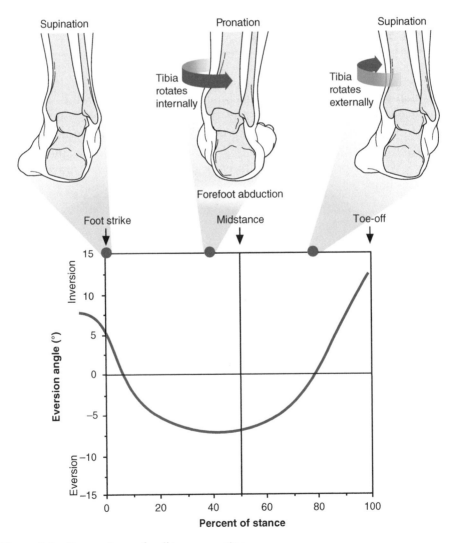

Figure 2.1   Stance phase of walking or running.

Pronation (figure 2.2*a*) is a combination of ankle dorsiflexion, rearfoot eversion (figure 2.3*a*), and forefoot abduction, and it occurs during the first half of stance (the cushioning, or eccentric, phase). The reverse movement is **supination** (figure 2.2*b*) which the foot moves back toward after heel-lift.

As seen in biomechanical graphs, the foot lands in a dorsiflexed position and then rapidly plantar flexes along a sagittal plane to bring the foot completely in contact with the ground (figure 2.4). Once the foot is completely on the ground, the ankle once again dorsiflexes as the **shank** moves anteriorly over the fixated foot; this dorsiflexion is a component of overall foot pronation. Coupled with this dorsiflexion motion along the frontal plane, as seen in figure 2.5, the foot everts from the instance of heel strike until approximately midstance, and the shank internally rotates during this same period (figure 2.6). So all three

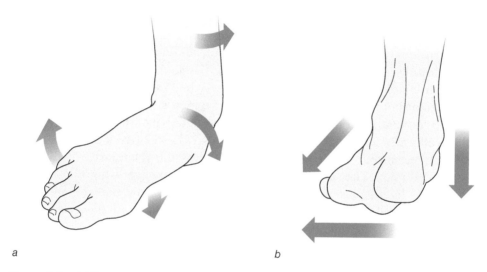

a   b

Figure 2.2 *(a)* Foot pronation and *(b)* supination.

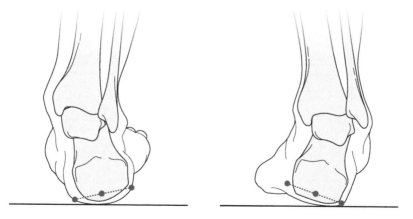

Figure 2.3 Rearfoot *(a)* eversion and *(b)* inversion.

components of overall foot pronation simultaneously occur from about 20% of stance until 50% of stance. Any frontal or transverse plane motion before 20% of stance occurs while the foot is not completely in contact with the ground and cannot be considered pronation based on the aforementioned definition. Foot pronation is a necessary and protective mechanism since it allows for

- impact forces to be attenuated over a longer period,
- the foot to accommodate uneven surfaces, and
- the foot to roll inward so that the first ray makes contact with the ground in preparation for resupination after heel lift.

 See online videos 2.1a to c for anterior, sagittal, and posterior views of typical foot mechanics during running.

With respect to the midfoot and associated deformation and forefoot abduction during the first half of stance, Dugan and Bhat (2005) investigated the 3-dimensional (3D) motion between rearfoot, midfoot, and forefoot segments in 18 healthy male subjects while walking barefoot. They reported that the contribution of midfoot motion was equivalent to 25% to 45% of the combined motions for both the forefoot and rearfoot segments and that total transverse plane (rotational) motion for the forefoot exceeded that of the rearfoot segment. Cornwall and McPoil (2004) also investigated the relative movement of the midfoot, measuring arch deformation and the possible relationship to dynamic rearfoot eversion. They concluded that the midfoot undergoes significant vertical and medial displacement during barefoot walking and that this motion is highly correlated with rearfoot eversion. Thus, lack of motion at the arch requires

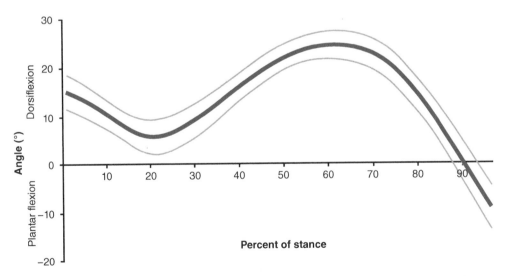

Figure 2.4 Biomechanical motion of ankle sagittal plane motion during the stance phase of running gait. A stance of 0% indicates heel strike, and a stance of 100% indicates toe-off.
Note: Blue line = mean; gray lines = ± 1 SD.

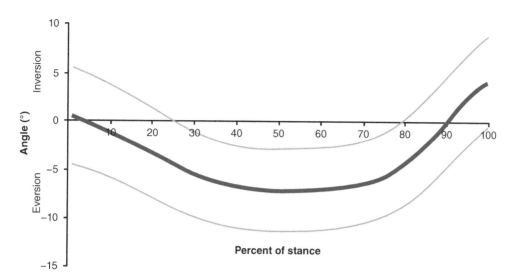

Figure 2.5 Biomechanical motion of ankle frontal plane motion during the stance phase of running gait. A stance of 0% indicates heel strike, and a stance of 100% indicates toe-off.
Note: Blue line = mean; gray lines = ± 1 SD.

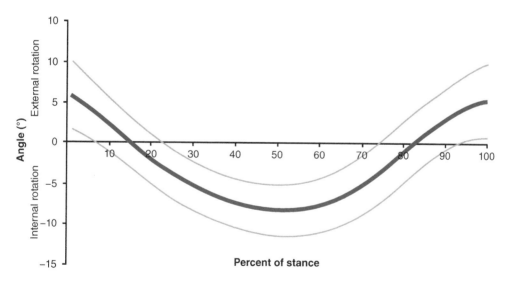

Figure 2.6 Biomechanical motion of tibial transverse plane motion during the stance phase of running gait. A stance of 0% indicates heel strike, and a stance of 100% indicates toe-off.
Note: Blue line = mean; gray lines = ± 1 SD.

greater relative rearfoot eversion to compensate, while midfoot hypermobility requires less relative rearfoot eversion. These results were supported by Hunt et al. (2001) and Leardini et al. (2007), who reported that the arch undergoes significant deformation during the first 74% of the stance phase of walking.

Rearfoot eversion influences lower extremity mechanics via tibial rotation (Macera et al. 1989; McClay and Manal 1997; Duffey et al. 2000; Waryasz and

McDermott 2008). During closed-chain pronation, when the calcaneus is fixed to the ground, it cannot abduct relative to the talus. Therefore, to obtain the transverse plane component of subtalar joint pronation, the talus adducts and medially rotates (Inman 1976; Lundberg et al. 1989). Due to the tight articulation of the ankle mortise, the tibia internally rotates as the talus adducts (see figure 2.7). During this cushioning phase of stance, the knee joint flexes, which is also associated with tibial internal rotation (Inman 1976; Lundberg et al. 1989). During gait, there is a direct relationship between the degree of pronation and internal tibial rotation for runners who exhibit a heel–toe footfall pattern (Dugan and Bhat 2005). Because there is normally more rearfoot eversion than tibial internal rotation, this ratio has been reported to vary between 1.2 and 1.8 (McClay and Manal 1997; Nawoczenski et al. 1998; Stacoff et al. 2000; Williams et al. 2001). In other words, every 1° of tibial internal rotation is associated with approximately 1.2° to 1.8° of rearfoot eversion.

Researchers (Subotnick 1995; Hreljac 2004) suggested that a higher level of pronation is favorable during running if it falls within so-called normal physiological limits and does not continue beyond midstance. After midstance, it is necessary for the foot to become more rigid and supinate (tibia and talus externally rotate and rearfoot inverts) in

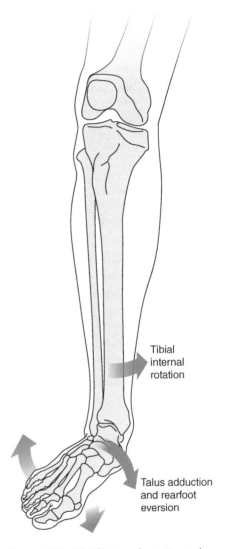

Tibial internal rotation

Talus adduction and rearfoot eversion

Figure 2.7 Tibial internal rotation, talus adduction, and knee flexion during the stance phase of gait.

preparation for toe-off (Inman 1976; Lundberg et al. 1989) (figure 2.7). Severe over-pronators, or runners who exhibit **prolonged pronation**, may be at an increased risk of injury due to the potentially large torques generated in the lower extremity and the subsequent increase in internal tibial rotation (figure 2.7) (Messier and Pittala 1988; Messier et al. 1991; McClay and Manal 1997; Hamill et al. 1999; Cheung and Ng 2007). This situation results in a mechanical dilemma at the knee because knee extension begins around midstance and must be accompanied by tibial external rotation to maintain joint congruity. However, since the tibia is internally rotated with the rearfoot, the hip must excessively internally rotate to maintain proper knee and patellofemoral joint position. The compensatory hip internal rotation may alter normal patellofemoral alignment and cause excessive contact pressures on the patella. This excessive pressure eventually leads to cartilage breakdown and anterior knee pain.

 See the online videos for examples of runners with
- **Excessive rearfoot eversion (video 2.2)**
- **Prolonged rearfoot eversion (video 2.3)**
- **Excessive eversion velocity (videos 2.4a and b)**

ATYPICAL FOOT MECHANICS AND INJURY

Excessive rearfoot eversion, eversion velocity, and time to maximum eversion have been implicated as contributing factors to overuse running injuries (Clarke et al. 1983; McKenzie et al. 1985; James and Jones 1990; Messier et al. 1991; Rolf 1995; James 1998). However, minimal and conflicting experimental evidence exists about whether excessive rearfoot eversion is a contributing factor in the etiology of injuries and, unfortunately, the majority of most studies are cross-sectional in design.

One study (Messier and Pittala 1988), which partially supported the speculation of a cause-and-effect relationship between rearfoot eversion and injury, reported that groups of injured runners exhibited greater peak rearfoot eversion and had greater maximum eversion velocities than a group of uninjured control subjects. The results were evident in the group of subjects who suffered from medial tibial stress syndrome (MTSS). Viitasalo and Kvist (1983) reported similar results when comparing runners with MTSS to uninjured control subjects during barefoot running. However, contradictory results were found in another study (Hreljac et al. 2000), in which runners who had never sustained an overuse injury exhibited greater eversion velocity and greater rearfoot inversion angle at heel strike than runners who had previously sustained an overuse injury. Yet another study compared runners who suffered from PFPS to a group of uninjured control subjects (Messier et al. 1991) and no differences in any rearfoot variables were found. Thus, no definitive answer is available based on these retrospective cross sectional design studies.

Unfortunately, only two prospective studies have been conducted to investigate the link between foot mechanics and overuse injuries. Willems et al. (2006) and Willems et al. (2007) evaluated lower-leg pain in a group of 400 young, physically active individuals. Plantar pressure measurements and 3D rearfoot kinematic data were collected and subjects were followed over a 9-month period. Seventy-five injured runners were identified and their data were compared to 167 non-injured runners. The injured runners exhibited significantly greater time to peak rearfoot eversion, increased medial foot pressure, and increased inversion velocity during the second half of stance as compared with controls. Thus, these data provide evidence that excessive foot pronation mechanics are contributing factors in the etiology of running-related injuries. However, in contrast, Thijs et al. (2007) examined gait-related risk factors for patellofemoral pain in a group of 84 officer cadets over the course of a 6-week basic military training period using plantar pressure measurements. Thirty-six cadets developed patellofemoral pain and exhibited a more inverted rearfoot position at heel strike and reduced eversion (greater lateral contact pressure) as compared with the control group.

Thus, the only two prospective studies conducted to date provide conflicting results as one study suggests excessive foot pronation is related to injury development while the other study suggests reduced foot pronation is related. Based on these data, and contradictory results from the various retrospective cross sectional studies outlined previously, no definitive answer can be put forth regarding potential running-related injury mechanisms and excessive foot pronation. As such, atypical foot biomechanics may not be the root cause, or rarely the sole factor, in understanding the etiology or in developing the subsequent treatment of any given lower extremity injury. Other factors, such as anatomical alignment, strength, and flexibility must also be considered.

 See online videos 2.5a and b for examples of a runner with reduced foot mechanics.

STRENGTH

When in a pronated position, the **subtalar** and **talocrural joints** are more mobile and require more muscle work to maintain stability compared to a supinated position. Several muscles are involved in this dynamic support, including but not limited to the tibialis posterior, peroneus longus, and tibialis anterior. The tibialis posterior is believed to play a key role in controlling rearfoot eversion (O'Connor and Hamill 2004; Pohl et al. 2010) and providing dynamic support across the midfoot and forefoot during the stance phase of gait (Thordarson et al. 1995; Kitaoka et al. 1997; Pohl et al. 2010). Furthermore, it has been postulated that when the tibialis posterior muscle is weak, greater rearfoot eversion is measured. However, the direct connection between reduced strength and altered biomechanics is difficult to discern based on a review of the current literature.

The proximal origin of tibialis posterior lies on the interosseous membrane and posterior surfaces of the tibia and fibula. The muscle has multiple distal insertions including the navicular tubercle, the plantar surface of the cuneiforms and cuboid, and bases of the second, third, and fourth metatarsals (figure 2.8) (Moore and Dalley 2005).

Biomechanical research conducted on patients with posterior tibialis tendon dysfunction (PTTD) while involving a fatigue protocol (Pohl et al. 2010; Ferber and Pohl 2011) highlights the importance of this muscle in controlling rearfoot, midfoot, and forefoot mechanics during gait (Rattanaprasert et al. 1999; Tome et

al. 2006; Ness et al. 2008). Two studies from our laboratory (Pohl et al. 2010; Ferber and Pohl 2011), based on a
tibialis posterior fatigue protocol and repeated bouts of
exercise, show that the force output from this muscle is
reduced by over 30%. For the fatigue protocol, subjects
were seated in a chair while their right foot was placed
in a custom-built device that allowed them to perform
concentric and eccentric foot adduction contractions
with adjustable resistance. Then with the ankle positioned in 20° plantar flexion, subjects performed sets
of 50 concentric and eccentric contractions at 50% of
maximal voluntary contraction (MVC) force through
a 30° range of motion. The subjects were allowed 10
seconds of rest between each set, and after every four
sets, maximum voluntary isometric force output was
measured again. The sets were continued until subjects'
isometric force output had dropped below 70% of the
pre-fatigue values or they were unable to complete two
consecutive sets.

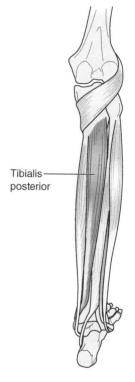

Tibialis posterior

Figure 2.8 Tibialis posterior.

Little to no change in rearfoot or forefoot kinematics
was observed as a result of the reduction in force output
(Pohl et al. 2010). Specifically, only a 0.7° increase in
peak rearfoot eversion was reported as statistically significant, but this change was smaller than the precision
error of a within-day gait analysis of 0.9°. Therefore,
the results were not clinically relevant, and it is pos-
sible that other muscles, such as the tibialis anterior, may have compensated for
the lack of tibialis posterior force production, thereby resulting in no change
in discrete kinematic variables. However, inspection of the data also revealed
that 24 out of 29 participants demonstrated an increase in peak rearfoot angle
following fatigue (ranging from 0.5° to 2.0°).

Despite these results not being statistically significant, there was a pattern
consistent enough to be of interest, and we decided to explore the data further.
Since such a consistent change was observed, it raises the question of what
other mechanisms and potential explanations can account for these systematic
changes. Thus, we reanalyzed the data based on **joint coupling** and **coupling
variability**. This analysis revealed increases in coupling motion of the shank
in the transverse plane and forefoot in the **sagittal plane** and **transverse plane**
relative to **frontal plane motion** of the rearfoot (Pohl et al. 2010). In addition,
an increase in joint coupling variability was measured between the shank and
rearfoot and between the rearfoot and forefoot during the fatigue condition. It
was concluded that once the tibialis posterior muscle was fatigued, fewer muscles
were functioning to achieve a desired movement pattern, and alterations in joint
coupling and coupling variability resulted.

Based on the redundancy of the various muscles that serve to control frontal plane rearfoot and transverse plane tibial motion, a potential strategy for the foot may be to increase coupling variability to avoid injury when the function of some muscles is compromised. Therefore, it can be hypothesized that with a diminished ability of the tibialis posterior muscle to produce a vigorous contraction, a concomitant reduction in joint contact force and a resulting increase in joint coupling variability could result. In other words, the reduced function of the tibialis posterior muscle after fatigue could result in less control of the ankle joint movement since fewer muscles are functioning to achieve a movement pattern that minimizes injury potential or pain while running.

Reduced force output from the tibialis posterior does not necessarily or automatically result in a greater peak rearfoot eversion angle. However, lack of strength from the tibialis posterior could be the root cause of several different musculoskeletal injuries based on its interrelationship with other muscles and the aforementioned changes in coupling among the rearfoot, tibia, and forefoot. For example, the tibialis posterior and soleus are the two primary stabilizing muscles at the ankle joint (O'Connor and Hamill 2004). Collectively, these two muscles have two main functions: to minimize torsional forces at the ankle and lower leg and to control rearfoot eversion during the stance phase of gait. In addition, the tibialis posterior muscle attaches to multiple sites on the plantar surface of the foot (figure 2.8) and thus serves to dynamically support the medial longitudinal arch. If the tibialis posterior muscle cannot produce adequate force, greater stress is placed on the soleus muscle to accomplish the aforementioned tasks, which partially explains the development of Achilles tendinopathy and overall calf pain and tightness. In addition, weakness of the tibialis posterior directly increases stress to the plantar fascia, which serves to statically support the arch of the foot and can help explain the development of plantar fasciitis.

ANATOMICAL ALIGNMENT

While excessive rearfoot motion during gait has received much attention in the literature, its relationship with anatomical structure remains unclear. Overall, one cannot assume that there is a direct relationship between anatomical foot structure and dynamic foot biomechanics. For instance, one study reported that a greater **standing rearfoot angle** was associated with greater measures of rearfoot eversion during walking (Donatelli et al. 1999). In contrast, Cornwall and McPoil (2004) showed no relationship between static measures and dynamic rearfoot motion.

The conflicting findings may be due to neglecting the role of muscular support when studying the relationship between the static and dynamic behavior of the rearfoot. For example, subjects with pronated foot posture have been shown to exhibit increased tibialis posterior activity as compared with those with a normal foot structure (Murley et al. 2009). Individuals with structural deficiencies, such as excessive **rearfoot valgus**, may rely more heavily on muscular contributions to control rearfoot kinematics during gait. Thus, it might be expected that these subjects would undergo greater changes in rearfoot kinematics after fatiguing exercise of a major invertor muscle. However, based on the literature, this assumption is wrong.

In the aforementioned tibialis posterior fatigue studies, there was a poor relationship between the standing rearfoot angle and changes in rearfoot walking kinematics following fatigue. Therefore, subjects who had greater standing rearfoot valgus angles did not rely more on tibialis posterior to control rearfoot motion during walking (Pohl et al. 2010). These results suggest that the anatomical structure of the foot is not associated with an increase in muscular activity required to maintain normal foot kinematics during gait. However, other muscles may have compensated for reduced force output from the tibialis posterior. Therefore, it is possible that compensation strategies masked the true relationship between anatomical structure and tibialis posterior contribution, which explains the increase in rearfoot, tibia, and forefoot coupling variability. Moreover, several structural aspects of the foot were not included in the previously mentioned studies, such as forefoot alignment, which are important to consider.

Another structural measure to consider is forefoot orientation relative to the rearfoot. Clinically, **forefoot varus** contributes to decreasing the medial longitudinal arch and therefore resembles **pes planus** (flat feet). During the stance phase of running the midfoot and forefoot are completely pronated in an attempt to bring the first metatarsal head in contact with the ground (figure 2.2a). The forefoot varus position necessitates greater rearfoot eversion to bring the first digit toward the ground to act as a rigid lever in preparation for toe-off (figure 2.9).

In contrast, **forefoot valgus** contributes to increasing the medial longitudinal arch and therefore resembles **pes cavus** (high arches). During the stance phase

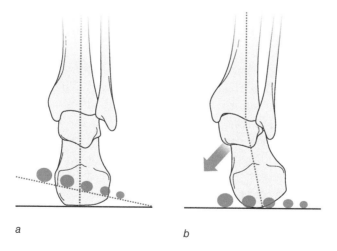

a   b

Figure 2.9 Example of the relationship between forefoot varus, midfoot collapse, and rearfoot eversion during pronation. With (a) forefoot varus, the first metatarsophalangeal (MTP) joint is rotated upwards, relative to a neutral rearfoot, and a (b) rearfoot valgus position is necessary to bring all metatarsals in contact with the ground.

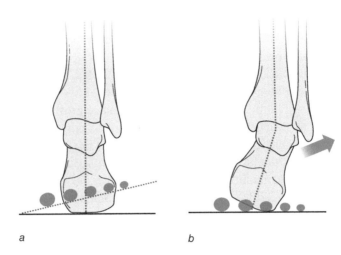

Figure 2.10 Example of the midfoot valgus, rearfoot inversion, and lack of midfoot collapse during pronation. With (*a*) forefoot valgus, the fifth MTP is rotated upwards, relative to a neutral rearfoot, and a (*b*) **rearfoot varus** position is necessary to bring all metatarsals in contact with the ground.

of running this places the rearfoot in a more supinated (reduced eversion or an inverted position) position so that the lateral aspect of the foot is in contact with the ground (figure 2.10).

A study by Buchanan and Davis (2005) measured forefoot varus and valgus and standing rearfoot angle on 51 individuals. Forefoot angles were obtained with the subject prone on the table and their foot in a neutral position. Varus (positive degrees), neutral (0°), or valgus (negative degrees) was measured as the angle between the bisection of the calcaneus and an imaginary perpendicular line drawn through the metatarsal heads (figure 2.11). Rearfoot angles were obtained with the subject standing and measured as the angle between the bisection of the lower one third of the leg and the bisection of the calcaneus.

The authors reported that a forefoot varus angle was present in 92% and a forefoot valgus angle was present in 8% of the cases. These results were also in agreement with data reported by Donatelli et al. (1999) and Garbalosa et al. (1994). Buchanan and Davis (2005) also examined the relationship between these two anatomical measures and reported a strong relationship. Specifically, a rearfoot valgus standing posture is most likely associated with a forefoot varus alignment, whereas a rearfoot varus standing posture is associated with a forefoot valgus alignment.

FLEXIBILITY

While there is limited research concerning the interrelationship between tissue flexibility and overall foot biomechanics, first ray mobility has been examined with respect to rearfoot motion. Cornwall and McPoil (2004) conducted a study

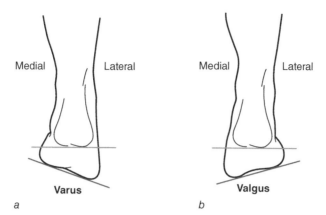

Figure 2.11 Forefoot angle measurement in prone relative to rearfoot angle in standing for *(a)* forefoot varus and *(b)* forefoot valgus.

to determine whether hypo- or hypermobility of the first ray influences rearfoot eversion during walking. Static measure of first ray mobility in 82 individuals (N = 164 feet) was measured and then classified as being hypomobile (n = 31), normal (n = 111), or hypermobile (n = 22). It was reported that a hypomobile first ray resulted in significantly more rearfoot eversion than those with either normal or hypermobile first rays. Thus, with a hypomobile first ray, greater rearfoot eversion is necessary to achieve overall foot pronation and should be considered when quantifying typical and atypical foot pronation mechanics. It is also interesting to note that the 82 subjects involved in this study were the same 82 subjects involved in a previous study that measured rearfoot standing posture, which found no correlation to rearfoot mechanics (Cornwall and McPoil 2004). A combined analysis of rearfoot standing posture and first ray mobility could have provided a more comprehensive understanding of rearfoot eversion biomechanics than the isolated analysis conducted.

Finally, adequate gastrocnemius and soleus flexibility is a critical component for proper foot biomechanics. Specifically, since **talocrural joint** dorsiflexion is a component of overall foot pronation, reduced relative motion between the gastrocnemius and soleus muscles can result in reduced ankle dorsiflexion and knee extension (You et al. 2009). Since the gastrocnemius muscle crosses the knee and ankle joints, reduced gastrocnemius muscle flexibility also influences the kinematic patterns of the lower extremities during gait. This study (You et al. 2009) reported that gastrocnemius tightness, defined as less than 12° for passive dorsiflexion with the knee extended, resulted in several different compensatory patterns including greater hip and knee flexion angles at the time of maximal ankle dorsiflexion and reduced knee energy absorption but increased ankle energy absorption during the first half of stance. Thus, reduced calf muscle flexibility can result in a redistribution of forces throughout the lower extremity and must be considered when trying to understand injury etiology.

SUMMARY

Based on an examination of various clinical factors, one can begin to draw conclusions on the expected biomechanics of the foot. For example, with a greater standing rearfoot eversion angle, low arch position, excessive forefoot varus position, weakness in the tibialis posterior muscle, and a hypermobile first ray, an excessively pronating foot with respect to greater rearfoot eversion and arch deformation is expected. In contrast, with a typical standing rearfoot eversion angle, typical arch height, a slight forefoot varus position, adequate strength in the tibialis posterior muscle, and a typical first ray position and mobility, a typically pronating foot is expected. Moreover, with only one variable outside of normal limits, an atypical pronation movement pattern would not be expected. It takes the combination of several factors to produce an excessive peak rearfoot eversion or prolonged time to peak rearfoot eversion (prolonged pronation). In the next chapter, we extend the discussion of foot biomechanics to consider footwear selection for runners.

CHAPTER

3

Footwear Selection

Although very few overuse running injuries have an established etiology, the fact that over 80% of these injuries occur at or below the knee suggests that there may be some common mechanisms. The capacity to prevent such injuries is currently limited, with training advice and footwear selection forming the mainstays. Thus, the prescription of the correct running shoe is considered a crucial and highly valued skill. Unfortunately, a systematic review by Richards et al. (2009) concluded that "the prescription of [pronation control] shoe type to distance runners is not evidence-based" (p. 161). Moreover, Ryan et al. (2011) conducted a study in which runners were randomized to receive a neutral, stability, or motion control running shoe. It was reported that prescribing motion control shoes incorrectly, without proper justification or rationale, is potentially injurious.

We discuss the research behind running shoes and begin to develop a basis for objective methods for footwear prescription. Then we place this method within the framework of mechanics, strength, flexibility, and alignment. Finally, we provide an overview of how running barefoot alters running mechanics and discuss the influence of foot orthotic devices.

OVERVIEW OF RUNNING SHOES

Overall, there are three categories of footwear: neutral, stability, and motion control. A neutral running shoe provides cushioning and less foot control than its motion control counterpart (figure 3.1). It typically has softer and more shock-absorbent material in the posterolateral aspect of the heel to better cushion at heel strike and provide a better transition from the heel to the midfoot and toe. A **neutral shoe** also has an elevated heel with a drop in height between the heel and toe typically around 10 to 12 mm.

This type of shoe is for those who exhibit typical foot structure, mobility, alignment, and foot pronation mechanics. It can also be prescribed for those individuals who exhibit a pes cavus, hypomobile midfoot and forefoot, a forefoot valgus alignment, and reduced pronation (supination) mechanics because they need greater cushioning in light of their intrinsically rigid foot. A neutral shoe's design is around a **semicurved last** or **curved last**, which is the amount of curvature from heel to toe relative to the amount of **foot flare** (figures 3.2 and 3.3) (see the Shoe Fitting section for a full description of shoe last).

A **stability shoe** has some component of pronation control material, and that material is generally placed near the middle or arch of the shoe (figure 3.4). Pronation control material implies that the shoe has a multiple-density midsole, typically with a second high-density foam on the medial aspect of the shoe, to reduce the rate of compression and control the amount of maximum foot pronation along that portion of the shoe. Therefore, the high-density foam provides less cushioning than a neutral shoe. In the case of a stability shoe, the placement of higher density foam is typically near the arch and will serve to minimize arch deformation and indirectly limit peak rearfoot eversion. A stability shoe is generally constructed around a semicurved last.

A stability shoe is designed for those individuals who do not excessively pronate but have some foot characteristics, in combination with their overall

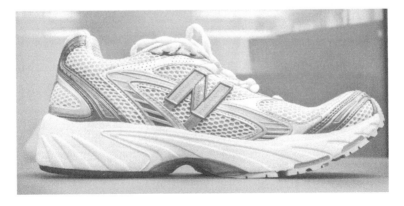

Figure 3.1 Neutral shoe. Note the consistent foam throughout the entire shoe, which provides for greater cushioning.

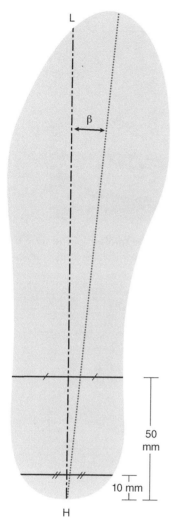

Figure 3.2 Calculating the last of a shoe. Perpendicular lines are drawn at 10 mm and 50 mm from the posterior aspect of the shoe (position H) and an orthogonal line (L) drawn to create the long axis of the rearfoot. A second line is then drawn from H to the center of the forefoot and the angle (β) subtended by the line connecting the two lines is the measure of the shoe's last.

Reprinted, by permission, from R.S. Goonetilleke and A. Luximon, 1999, "Foot flare and foot axis," *Human Factors: The Journal of the Human Factors and Ergonomics Society* 41: 596.

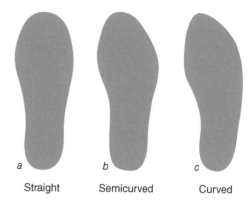

Figure 3.3 The basic shapes of running shoes with *(a)* straight, *(b)* semicurved, and *(c)* curved last.

foot mechanics, that place increased pronatory and torsional forces on their foot and lower leg while running. For example, a greater than typical forefoot varus alignment, a hypermobile first ray, or a rearfoot that exhibits slightly greater passive rearfoot eversion range of motion than considered normal in combination or alone may necessitate a stability shoe.

A **motion control shoe** typically has a significant amount of pronation control material and often has some type of nondeformable material, such as a plastic plug, placed on the posteromedial aspect of the shoe (figure 3.5). The high-density foam typically extends into the rearfoot of the shoe and is meant to limit excessive arch deformation and excessive rearfoot eversion. This type of shoe has a **straight-lasted** construction.

Obviously, because of the considerable amount of high-density foam, there is significantly less cushioning than a neutral shoe and somewhat less than a stability shoe. A motion control shoe is for those individuals with a foot structure consisting of excessive rearfoot eversion biomechanics (see chapter 2), a greater than normal forefoot varus alignment, pes planus, and hypermobility of the first ray and midfoot.

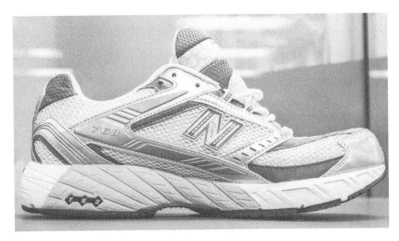

Figure 3.4 Stability shoe. Note the high-density foam near the midfoot of the shoe that limits midfoot collapse and provides less cushioning as compared with a neutral shoe.

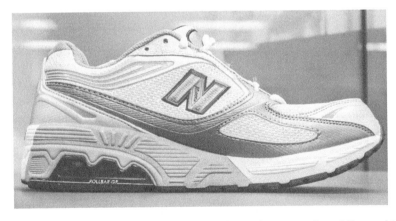

Figure 3.5 Motion control shoe. Note the high-density foam near the midfoot, which limits midfoot collapse, and the plastic plug at the posterior aspect of the shoe, which limits rearfoot eversion. They provide less cushioning than a stability shoe or especially a neutral shoe.

FOOTWEAR RESEARCH FINDINGS

The existing literature has generally investigated different components of the shoe in isolation to determine their effects on foot and lower-leg kinematics during running. The primary components that have been investigated are differences in midsole hardness, the differences in heel flare, and the effects of pronation control material.

Overall, mixed results have been reported when alterations in midsole hardness have been investigated. For example, it has been reported that softer shoes allow greater rearfoot eversion (Clarke et al. 1983; De Wit et al. 1995) but result in no differences in magnitude or loading rate of ankle and knee joint forces

(Nigg and Morlock 1987). Research has also reported no differences in peak tibial acceleration regardless of changes in midsole hardness, while others have reported increases in midsole hardness result in small changes in sagittal plane ankle kinematics (Hardin et al. 2004; Nigg and Morlock 1987). Another study found nonsystematic or subject specific changes in knee flexion, ankle plantar flexion velocity, and maximum rearfoot eversion across shoes with different midsole properties (Kersting and Bruggemann 2006).

These same conflicting results have been reported with respect to changes in the amount of heel flare. In two separate studies, decreasing the amount of heel flare was shown to affect only rearfoot eversion angle at touchdown but not rearfoot eversion excursion or maximum eversion angle, both of which occur during midstance while running (Nigg et al. 1987; Nigg and Morlock 1987). While in another study, greater heel flare allowed increased rearfoot eversion and eversion excursion (Clarke et al. 1983). Thus, altering individual components of a shoe does not produce a consistent change in foot, ankle, or leg kinematics, but rather small and non-systematic changes.

The most logical explanation for these conflicting results is that the aforementioned studies investigated only individual components of a shoe and did not compare across shoe categories such as motion control versus neutral shoes. It has been reported that, compared with a neutral shoe, motion control shoes provide a more stable electrical activation pattern and higher fatigue resistance for the tibialis anterior and peroneus longus muscles after a fatiguing run (Cheung and Ng 2010). In meta-analysis of footwear-related studies, motion control shoes were reported to significantly reduce peak rearfoot eversion compared with a neutral shoe (Cheung et al. 2011). Furthermore, the control of rearfoot eversion when running in the motion control shoe was maintained even after the fatigue protocol as compared to the neutral shoe.

Interestingly, only one study has investigated the interaction between arch structure and shoe type (Butler et al. 2006). In this study, motion control shoes were matched to runners with a pes planus (flat feet) structure, while a neutral shoe was matched for a pes cavus (high arches) structure. The study involved running in both shoe conditions (Butler et al. 2006). For the pes planus runners, peak tibial internal rotation decreased when running in the motion control shoe and was increased in the neutral shoe over the course of a prolonged run. However, the magnitude of rearfoot eversion was the same regardless of the shoe worn by the pes planus runners. For the pes cavus runners, lower tibial shock was measured when running in the neutral shoe as compared to the motion control shoe. The authors concluded that when wearing the recommended shoe for arch structure, specific biomechanical characteristics were altered that could potentially reduce injury risk. However, the individuals involved in this study were at the extremes of arch structure and do not represent the typical population of runners. Moreover, other foot characteristics, such as rearfoot standing posture and first ray mobility, and the strength of the tibialis posterior muscle were not considered.

While this one study provides some evidence suggesting that an approach of fitting shoes based on anatomical structure may be effective, there is no other evidence within the literature to support this concept. First, there has been no research involving stability shoes compared with neutral or motion control shoes. Second, a systematic review by Richards et al. (2009) concluded that there is no evidence-based method for the prescription of

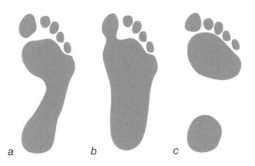

Figure 3.6 Wet test sample results for *(a)* normal, *(b)* pes planus, and *(c)* pes cavus foot structure.

shoe type to distance runners. Moreover, research investigating the prescription of footwear for new recruits based on plantar shape, a method analogous to the wet test (figure 3.6), found no reduction in injuries between the treatment group and control group during basic training (Knapik et al. 2009; Knapik, Brosch et al. 2010; Knapik, Spiess et al. 2010). Another study that randomly assigned shoes to individuals regardless of arch type found that there were more injuries in individuals with a motion control shoe even if they case matched, suggesting that motion control shoe prescription can potentially be injurious (Ryan et al. 2011). Thus, a more systematic, scientific, and objective approach must be utilized to place the proper foot within the proper shoe.

SHOE FITTING

Currently, there is no formula or standard algorithm for the basis of footwear selection. However, based on the research we can propose an approach based on foot structure, measures of forefoot orientation, arch height, and rearfoot standing posture. Other considerations, such as dynamic rearfoot motion, can be considered, but the accuracy of these measures is questionable and will be discussed in chapter 9.

For individuals with a forefoot varus angle (present in 92% of individuals), when the forefoot initially strikes the ground, the first ray is elevated relative to the fifth ray (see chapter 2 for more details). To place the first ray on the ground, the forefoot naturally adducts resulting in an inward foot-flare angle. These data are in agreement with Goonetilleke (1999) who traced and measured flare angles, finding a mean foot flare of 3° to 5°, which is approximately the amount of curvature (last) for a semicurved shoe. Thus, the vast majority of the population has an inward forefoot flare and should be fitted for a semicurved or a curved running shoe depending on the amount of forefoot varus.

When determining the curvature of the foot, the plantar silhouette can be measured similar to Goonetilleke (1999) or the amount of forefoot varus or valgus can be measured. Since Buchanan and Davis (2005) reported an average varus angle of 4.4° (± 3.4°), the following method can be used to determine the association between foot curvature and shoe last: Forefoot varus angles that fall within 1° and 8° optimally fit within a semicurved shoe, whereas forefoot varus angles greater than 8° necessitate a curve-lasted shoe. On the other hand, a forefoot valgus or a neutral forefoot orientation optimally fits within a straight-lasted shoe. It can also be assumed that a forefoot varus angle between 1° and 8° is associated with typical pronation mechanics and therefore functions best within a neutral shoe. The same rationale for shoe recommendation follows for a valgus forefoot since it exhibits reduced pronation or supination biomechanics. Thus, a valgus angle greater than 8° exhibits excessive pronation mechanics and necessitates a stability or motion control shoe.

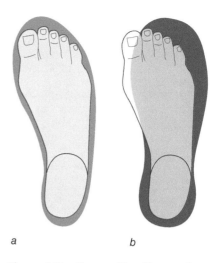

Figure 3.7 Flare and its effect on shoe fit. *(a)* A matching of a curve-lasted shoe and a curved foot. *(b)* Mismatch between a straight-lasted shoe and a curved foot.

As one example for considering foot curvature with respect to shoe last, consider that since motion control shoes are typically straight lasted, most feet (92%) will not fit properly and will be prone to atypical frictional forces (figure 3.7).

With respect to measuring arch height, it has been reported that visual assessment of the plantar surface is not accurate for determining low and high foot arches (Swedler et al. 2010). Moreover, the navicular drop test, in which the navicular tubercle is marked and the distance measured to the floor in both a sitting and standing position, has high levels of intrarater reliability but unacceptably poor levels of interrater reliability, suggesting that use of this measure among clinicians is not recommended (McPoil et al. 2008). New methods to assess arch height should be developed because of this and because of a lack of normative data from a cohort of healthy individuals.

In response, the arch height index (AHI) has been shown to be a valid and reliable method of measuring anatomical aspects of the arch (Butler et al. 2006). AHI is measured using a custom built arch height index measurement system. Two boards are placed under the foot, one under the calcaneus and one under the forefoot to allow the midfoot to achieve maximum deformation (figure 3.8). The measure of AHI is unitless and is defined as the ratio of dorsum height at 50% of total foot length, divided by the foot length from the back of the heel to the head of the first metatarsal, defined as the truncated foot length (Fields et al. 2010). Seated AHI is obtained with the participant seated, hips and knees flexed to 90°, and approximately 10% of total body weight on the foot. Standing AHI is obtained with the participant standing with equal weight on both feet. The AHI measurement has been deemed an appropriate measurement of static

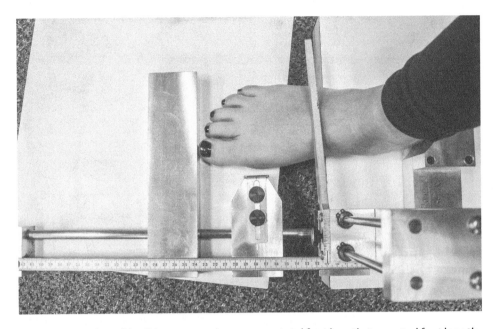

Figure 3.8 Adjustable sliders are used to measure total foot length, truncated foot length, and dorsal height at 50% of total foot length.

foot structure because its very good to excellent reliability has been previously demonstrated in the literature (Williams and McClay 2000; Butler et al. 2006).

Butler et al. (2006) reported that the mean AHI for a group of recreational runners was 0.340 to 0.363 ± 0.030 for sitting and 0.340 ± 0.030 for standing. The AHI between genders was similar. Thus, if the AHI value for a runner falls within these values for both sitting and standing, they have a typical arch structure and therefore optimally fit within a neutral shoe. A low AHI value indicates a pes planus structure and therefore necessitates a stability or motion control shoe, whereas a high AHI value indicates a pes cavus structure and thus is best suited with a neutral shoe.

McPoil et al. (2009) used a similar approach by measuring arch height with a digital caliper and reported normative data for the left and right feet of 211 female and 134 male participants. These authors reported excellent within and between session reliability values ranging from 0.97 to 0.99 for various weight-bearing and non-weight-bearing foot measures. Moreover, they reported that the average amount of arch deformation during weight bearing, compared with sitting measures, was between 1.19 cm and 1.35 cm for both males and females. Thus, if a clinician does not have access to an AHI device, a simple digital caliper can also be used to measure arch deformation.

Finally, measures of standing-rearfoot posture can also be used to determine the optimal shoe. Cornwall and McPoil (2004) reported a measure of 6.3° (±4.0°) for static rearfoot–shank angle from 82 individuals. Sobel et al. (1999) reported a similar measure of 6.07° (±2.71°) for 88 adults, while Kendall et al. (2008)

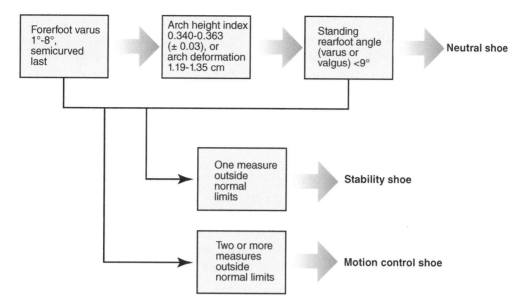

Figure 3.9 Flow chart of various anatomical foot measurements and their relationship to determination of a neutral shoe. Note that our approach is that if any measure is outside of normal limits, a stability shoe is recommended. If any two measures are outside of normal limits, a motion control shoe is recommended.

reported an average angle of 6.10° (±2.58°) in 221 runners. Based on these large samples, a static rearfoot–shank angle of 6° (±3°) could be considered normal and another appropriate measure for determining the optimal shoe. Measures of rearfoot valgus between 3° and 9° should be considered typical and function best within a neutral shoe. Similarly, valgus angles less than 3° or a rearfoot varus orientation (negative values) is associated with a supination biomechanical pattern and thus necessitate a neutral shoe as well. Valgus angles in excess of 9° would therefore necessitate a stability or motion control shoe.

In summary, the flow-chart in figure 3.9 may be useful in determining the proper shoe based on foot structure. However, please note that there is no scientific evidence to support the differentiation between stability and motion control shoes. In fact, no published research has investigated the potential biomechanical differences between these two shoe types. Therefore, the approach we take is that if any two measures indicate that a stability shoe is optimal, and the forefoot valgus orientation is in excess of 8°, indicating a straight-lasted foot, we suggest that a motion control shoe may be indicated as the optimal shoe.

BAREFOOT RUNNING

Barefoot running, or running in a minimalist shoe, has received increasing attention within the popular media over the past several years. However, one must first realize that barefoot running is not new to elite runners, with Abebe

Bikila winning gold in the 1960 Olympic marathon while running barefoot and Zola Budd setting the world record for the 5000 m at the 1984 Olympic games. The first research study published was in 1987 (Robbins and Hanna 1987). Since then, multiple studies have been conducted to understand the potential alterations in running mechanics when running barefoot. However, it is important to note that, to date, there is no research that either supports or refutes the injury preventative aspects of running barefoot that marketing campaigns and advertisements promote. There is only research to confirm that running barefoot is different than running shod.

While looking at the effects of running in shoes compared with running barefoot, it has been reported that running barefoot, or even running with a forefoot strike as opposed to a rearfoot strike, results in decreased stride length; increased **stride rate**; decreased range of motion at the ankle, knee, and hips; and a more plantar flexed ankle position at ground contact (De Wit et al. 2000; Divert et al. 2005; Lieberman et al. 2010). Moreover, Kerrigan et al. (2009) reported a 54% decrease in the hip rotational forces, a 36% decrease in knee flexion forces, and a 38% decrease in frontal plane knee forces when running barefoot compared with running in shoes.

While these results appear impressive, a closer inspection reveals that there is no clear answer about whether barefoot running is injury preventative or causative. For example, by decreasing stride length, and increasing stride rate, more steps are taken per kilometer. For the average runner running a marathon, this would result in 1,280 more steps to finish the race but only two minutes less of total foot contact time over a 3 hr, 20 min time compared to running shod. The increased numbers of steps and increased repetitions of maximum vertical loading when running barefoot (or with a forefoot strike pattern) could be injury-causative. On the other hand, 36% to 54% less force at the hip and knees for every step could be injury-preventative. Moreover, based on mechanical properties of the Achilles tendon (Konsgaard et al. 2011) and when considering that a forefoot strike pattern forces the heel downwards shortly after contact with the ground (Kerrigan et al. 2009; Lieberman et al. 2010), each step taken when running barefoot results in 59% of the force needed to rupture the Achilles tendon. The increased tensile loading of the Achilles tendon could result in tendinopathy, a gastrocnemius, or soleus muscle strain.

In summary, while research has been done on how barefoot running alters an individual's mechanical patterns and joint loading, no studies have been conducted on whether injury rates or specific injuries are reduced compared with shod running. Considering the complexity of the etiology of running injuries, changing one parameter such as footwear or even eliminating shoes altogether and completely altering the mechanical pattern cannot eliminate the occurrence or potential for musculoskeletal injuries. In fact, rapid alterations in one kinematic running pattern place a runner at risk for injury. Finally, considering that the magnitude of force applied to the system, a runner's mass, does not substantially change whether barefoot or shod, the changes in mechanics attributed to running barefoot or running with a forefoot strike would simply result in the impact force being redistributed elsewhere within the body. Thus, while barefoot running may result in a reduction of some injuries, such as to the knee and hip, we are likely to see an increase in other injuries, such as to the metatarsals, plantar fascia, and Achilles tendon. Future research will help answer these questions.

ORTHOTIC DEVICES AND FOOT MECHANICS

Foot orthotics have been shown to be efficacious for the treatment of running-related musculoskeletal injuries (Eggold 1981; Kilmartin and Wallace 1994). In terms of pain relief, success rates between 70% and 90% have been cited (Eggold 1981; Blake and Denton 1985; Gross et al. 1991; Landorf and Keenan 2000), and on average foot orthotics have a success rate of between 70% to 80% in the treatment of chronic knee injuries (James et al. 1978; Donatelli et al. 1988; Saxena and Haddad 2003). Donatelli et al. (1988) assessed the effects of semirigid plastic or fiberglass orthotics through a post-treatment survey. They reported that most patients experienced reduced pain after treatment, and 90% of those patients treated only with foot orthotics exhibited a reduction in pain and symptoms. James et al. (1978) used soft and rigid orthotics for runners with patellofemoral pain syndrome and other knee injuries and reported that 78% of those treated showed positive results. Saxena and Haddad (2003) used semiflexible molded orthotics for the treatment of knee pain and reported that 76% of the patients had reduced pain. In addition, a case study using thermoplastic orthotics for a patient with patellofemoral pain syndrome also showed reduction in pain with orthotic intervention (Way 1999). It has also been reported that 53% to 83% of patients continue to wear their orthotic devices even after their symptoms have been resolved (Donatelli et al. 1988; Moraros and Hodge 1993). Thus, these results strongly suggest that foot orthotics are effective in the treatment of overuse injury.

However, while the clinical efficacy of orthotic devices is widely documented, the mechanism behind that success is not well understood (Eggold 1981; Blake and Denton 1985; Gross et al. 1991; Landorf and Keenan 2000). Many biomechanical and electromyographic (EMG) investigations have been conducted to understand the alterations in lower-extremity kinematics, kinetics, and muscle EMG when running in an orthotic device. From a biomechanical perspective, foot orthotics have been hypothesized to control some aspects of rearfoot mechanics, such as peak eversion, eversion velocity or eversion excursion, and tibial internal rotation, but any changes are relatively small (Inman 1976; Bates et al. 1979; Smith et al. 1986; Donatelli et al. 1988; Lundberg et al. 1989; Novick and Kelley 1990; Baitch et al. 1991; Eng and Pierrynowski 1993; McCulloch et al. 1993; Brown et al. 1995; Nawoczenski et al. 1995; McPoil and Cornwall 2000; Stacoff et al. 2000; Mundermann et al. 2003a; Nester et al. 2003; MacLean et al. 2006). Mills et al. (2010) conducted a systematic review of 22 papers and meta-analysis of the scientific literature pertaining to the role of orthotics with different combinations of posting, molding, and density. These authors concluded that posted, nonmolded orthotics systematically reduced peak rearfoot eversion by approximately 2° and reduced tibial internal rotation by approximately 1° in noninjured cohorts. In contrast, only a few of the other aforementioned hypothetical mechanisms have been supported in the scientific literature. Thus, we can conclude that orthotics control rearfoot eversion but only to a small degree.

The studies investigating the effect of foot orthotic devices on ankle and knee joint moments and muscle EMG have reported conflicting and mixed results (Crenshaw et al. 2000; Mundermann et al. 2003a; Mundermann et al. 2003b; Nester et al. 2003; Nigg et al. 2003; Williams et al. 2003). Most of these studies used healthy, noninjured subjects to understand how an orthotic device functions to maintain or restore normal kinematics and kinetics of the foot, ankle, and lower leg. Unfortunately, only a handful of studies investigating the effect of orthotics on joint mechanics have included injured populations.

In addition, several studies have used either noncustom orthotics (wedges, cork inserts, prefabricated devices) (Bates et al. 1979; Rodgers and Leveau 1982; Milgrom et al. 1985; Smith et al. 1986; Gross et al. 1991; van Mechelen 1992; Eng and Pierrynowski 1993; Brown et al. 1995; Klingman et al. 1997; Nigg et al. 1999; Way 1999; Crenshaw et al. 2000; Hreljac et al. 2000; McPoil and Cornwall 2000; Neptune et al. 2000; Stacoff et al. 2000; Nigg et al. 2003; Saxena and Haddad 2003; Finestone et al. 2004) while only a few have investigated custom foot orthotics (Blake and Denton 1985; Blake 1986; Donatelli et al. 1988; Novick and Kelley 1990; Baitch et al. 1991; Tomaro and Burdett 1993; Nawoczenski et al. 1995; Hung and Gross 1999; Nawoczenski and Ludewig 1999; Rose et al. 2002; Mundermann et al. 2003a; Mundermann et al. 2003b; Nester et al. 2003; Williams et al. 2003; Ferber et al. 2005; MacLean et al. 2006; Mundermann et al. 2006).

Unfortunately, the majority of these studies have focused on rearfoot mechanics, producing varying results. Most orthotic devices have some type of arch support that either conforms to the shape of the medial longitudinal arch or functions to control arch deformation (Ferber 2007). Thus, it has been hypothesized that orthotics may function to minimize strain to the plantar fascia tissue through arch control (Neufeld and Cerrato 2008; Rosenbloom 2011). Moreover, Williams et al. (2003) suggested that orthotic devices could influence midfoot kinematics possibly by minimizing arch motion during running. However, only one study has investigated whether orthotics, either custom-made or semicustom in design, alter midfoot kinematics.

We conducted a study to determine changes in multisegment foot biomechanics during shod walking with and without an orthotic device (Ferber and Benson 2011). We chose to investigate a semicustom orthotic device that incorporates a heat-molding process to further understand if the molding process would significantly alter rearfoot or midfoot kinematics and plantar fascia strain compared with no orthotic. The findings indicate that semicustom molded orthotics reduce plantar fascia strain by 35% compared with walking without an orthotic. However, this particular device does not control peak rearfoot eversion, tibial internal rotation, or arch deformation. Finally, we found that heat molding the orthotic device does not have a measurable effect on the biomechanical variables compared to the nonmolded condition.

Therefore, while orthotics are considered a well-respected modality for the treatment of musculoskeletal injuries, the mechanism by which pain resolution occurs is not fully understood. Regardless, prescription of an orthotic device should follow similar principles as for a shoe. In other words, a thorough and objective approach to measurements of arch height, rearfoot eversion, and forefoot orientation along with objective measures of muscular strength, flexibility, and gait biomechanics will help in the prescription of an orthotic designed to control atypical foot mechanics.

SUMMARY

Matching a foot and shoe is a process that requires thought, scientific measurement, and rationale. Though the research on shoe selection is still incomplete, shoe selection based on foot structure and measures of forefoot orientation, arch height, and rearfoot standing posture can aid in injury prevention. With this information on the types of running shoes, a rationale and overall paradigm for shoe fitting using scientific methodology, and the scientific literature related to orthotics, we continue up the kinematic chain and discuss knee mechanics in chapter 4. We discuss some of the common running injuries runners sustain, discuss injury etiology, and most important, we have an in-depth discussion into the pathomechanics and interrelationships between strength, alignment, and flexibility.

Assessing Knee Mechanics

Now that we have considered several distal factors related to clinical gait analysis, including ankle and foot mechanics and footwear prescription, we move up the kinematic chain and discuss knee mechanics. We discuss biomechanical, strength, flexibility, and anatomical considerations using the most up-to-date research literature and practices.

BIOMECHANICS

During foot pronation, when the rearfoot is fixed to the ground, the calcaneus cannot abduct relative to the talus. Therefore, to obtain the transverse plane component of subtalar joint pronation, the talus adducts or medially rotates. Due to the tight articulation of the ankle mortise, the tibia internally rotates as the talus adducts. These mechanically linked motions occur during the first half of the stance phase of gait along with knee joint flexion, internal rotation, and adduction (figures 4.1-4.3). However, it is important to note that for most of the stance phase of gait, the knee undergoes only 4° to 6° of frontal plane motion and remains primarily in an inwardly collapsed position commonly called a genu valgum position (figure 4.4a). Rearfoot eversion, tibial internal rotation, knee flexion, and knee internal rotation (distal femur rotation on the tibia) occur relatively synchronously. During the second phase of gait, the propulsive phase of stance, these motions reverse, and the rearfoot inverts as the tibia and knee externally rotate when the knee extends.

 See online videos 4.1a to c for anterior, posterior, and sagittal views of typical knee mechanics during running.

Although the relative timing between the foot and the knee is nearly synchronous, minor variations in relative timing have been reported, and several investigations have reported relative asynchrony between these motions. For example, several authors have reported that peak rearfoot eversion occurs between 39% and 54% of stance while peak knee flexion occurs between 36% and 45% of stance (James et al. 1978; Van Woensel and Cavanaugh 1992; McClay

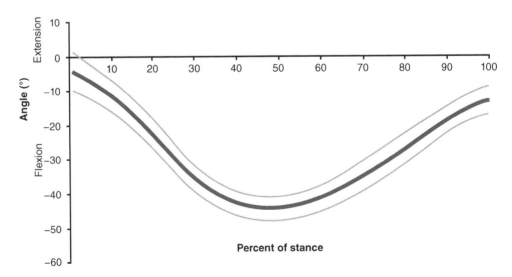

Figure 4.1 Biomechanical motion of knee sagittal plane motion during the stance phase of running gait. 0% of stance indicates heel strike, and 100% of stance indicates toe-off.

Note: Blue line = mean; gray lines = ± 1 SD.

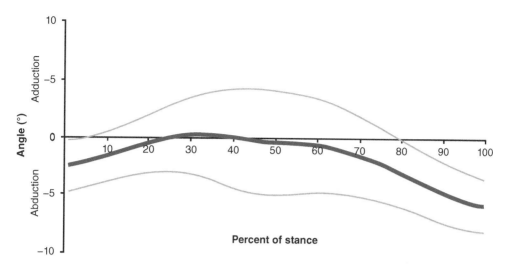

Figure 4.2 Biomechanical motion of knee frontal plane motion during the stance phase of running gait. 0% of stance indicates heel strike, and 100% of stance indicates toe-off.
Note: Blue line = mean; gray lines = ± 1 SD.

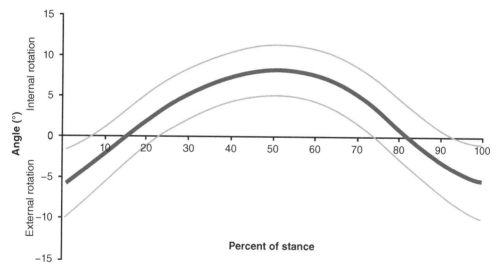

Figure 4.3 Biomechanical motion of knee transverse plane motion during the stance phase of running gait. 0% of stance indicates heel strike, and 100% of stance indicates toe-off.
Note: Blue line = mean; gray lines = ± 1 SD.

and Manal 1997; Stergiou et al. 1999; De Wit and De Clercq 2000). Moreover, inspection of figure 4.3 (knee rotation) in comparison with figure 2.6 (tibial rotation) shows that knee external rotation occurs in an asynchronous manner as compared to the tibia. Specifically, tibial external rotation begins near 50% of stance, coincident with rearfoot inversion, whereas knee external rotation occurs closer to 70% of stance. Previous studies have also measured the relative motion between rearfoot and knee in much the same way as was previously discussed in chapter 2 for the rearfoot and tibia.

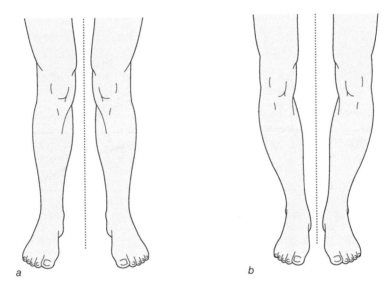

Figure 4.4 *(a)* Genu valgum and *(b)* genu varum.

The degree of coupling between the rearfoot and knee is influenced by the orientation of the subtalar joint axis in the sagittal plane. Using intracortical bone pins placed into the calcaneus and talus of cadaveric feet, Manter (1941) and Root et al. (1966) have reported that the orientation of the subtalar joint axis in the sagittal plane is approximately 41° to 42°, relative to the horizontal, with a range from 25° to 51°. If the subtalar joint axis were oriented at 45° in the sagittal plane, close to the average seen in these cadaver studies, one would expect equal amounts of rearfoot eversion and transverse plane tibial and knee internal rotation. However, as discussed in chapter 2, there is approximately 1.2° to 1.8° of rearfoot eversion for every degree of tibial internal rotation; the knee and tibia both exhibit less relative rotation than the frontal motion of the rearfoot. To explain this discrepancy, consider that the early studies of rearfoot and knee coupling involved measurements of cadaveric feet in a non-weight-bearing position, likely resulting in a higher orientation of the axis than is present during stance.

Lundberg et al. (1989) measured the orientation of the subtalar joint axis during stance in healthy subjects. Using an interesting approach, tantalum balls were injected into various bones of the foot, and relative 3D joint positions were measured using 2D biplanar radiographs. The authors reported an average orientation of subtalar joint axis of only 32° in the sagittal plane, ranging from 14° to 40°. Contrary to the earlier studies, but consistent with the biomechanical studies already discussed, these data suggest that the knee exhibits less relative rotation than the frontal motion of the rearfoot and less relative overall internal and external rotation than the tibia. Again, comparison of figure 4.3 and 2.6 support these findings and demonstrate these interrelationships. The clinical interpretation of the range of variation among individuals is that there is no norm and an individualized assessment must be performed for each patient to gain insight into the individual's specific biomechanical coupling pattern.

The rationale for understanding the timing of joint movements is based on the notion that asynchrony in these motions may result in injury. For example, Tiberio (1987) first proposed an interesting hypothetical mechanism for PFPS related to atypical or asynchronous joint coupling. He theorized that if the time to peak rearfoot eversion is prolonged and continues beyond midstance, tibial internal rotation would also be prolonged. These atypical mechanics result in a mechanical dilemma at the knee because knee extension begins around midstance and must be accompanied by tibial external rotation to maintain joint symmetry and congruity. However, since the tibia is continuing to internally rotate with the rearfoot, the femur must excessively internally rotate to obtain the relative knee external rotation needed for the second half of the stance phase. The result would be an increased amount of dynamic knee genu valgum (abduction), since knee internal rotation and abduction are mechanically linked, and an increased potential for other tissues to undergo atypical stress. Tiberio also went on to hypothesize that the compensatory femoral internal rotation may alter normal patellofemoral alignment and cause excessive contact pressures on the patella. This excessive pressure is thought to eventually lead to cartilage breakdown and anterior knee pain (Buchbinder et al. 1979; Cowan et al. 1996; Mizuno et al. 2001). However, one mechanism to resist or minimize the international rotation and concomitant patellar contact pressures would be adequate hip rotator strength (discussed in chapter 5) as well as those muscles responsible for controlling the knee.

 See online videos 4.2*a* to *d* for examples of a runner with excessive knee abduction (genu valgum).

STRENGTH

Many muscles cross the knee joint and serve to provide dynamic control and stabilization. Most pertinent to clinical gait analysis are the hamstring and quadriceps muscles. The hamstrings primarily function during the swing phase of gait to eccentrically control knee extension via control of the lower leg, or shank, in preparation for heel strike (figure 4.5*b*) (Chumanov et al. 2011). Thus, weakness of the hamstring musculature results in reduced **hip extension** at toe-off (figure 4.5*a*) to minimize the inertial motion of the shank and concomitant demand on the hamstring muscles during the swing phase. Moreover, since hip extension at toe-off is reduced, a reduced stride length and increased stride frequency will be measured on a step-by-step basis.

During the stance phase of gait, the hamstring muscles serve to stabilize the knee and maintain relative position of the tibia and femur with respect to translational motion. Pandy and Shelburne (1997) and Li et al. (1999) reported that

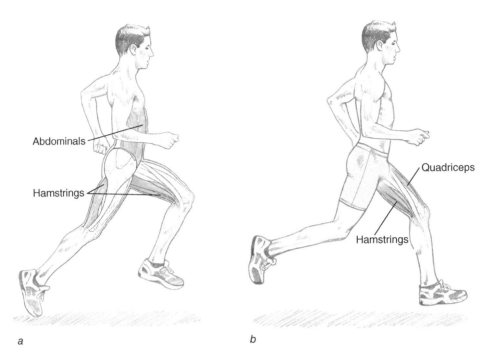

a   b

Figure 4.5 Muscle activity during the *(a)* toe-off and *(b)* forward swing phase of running gait.

during stance anterior tibial shear increases in magnitude from full extension to 15° flexion, then decreases as the knee flexes. The knee is near full extension at two points during stance: after heel strike (figure 4.6*a*) and near the end of stance (figure 4.6*b*). Thus, the hamstring muscles must serve as dynamic synergists to the anterior cruciate ligament and assist in reducing anterior tibial shear at these two points (Pandy and Shelburne 1997; Osternig et al. 2000). Weakness of the hamstring muscles allows for increased anterior tibial translation and increased shear forces to the anterior cruciate ligament and menisci of the knee joint during the first 20% of stance. Interestingly, the increase in shear forces is coupled with reciprocal action and down-regulation in force output from the quadriceps muscles (Osternig et al. 2000; Ferber et al. 2002b). The hamstring muscles, however, do less overall work during the stance phase of gait than the quadriceps (Anderson and Pandy 2003).

From foot flat to 20% of stance, the vasti muscles (medialis, lateralis, intermedius), along with the gluteus maximus and medius (discussed further in chapter 5) produce the majority of support and prevent the knee from collapsing against the downward pull of gravity and during knee flexion. Interestingly, rectus femoris, a biarticular muscle, contributes very little to overall support. In contrast, the uni-articular vasti muscles remain active throughout most of midstance until heel lift and, as previously discussed in chapter 2, generate nearly all support in late stance along with the soleus and gastrocnemius. All other muscles crossing the knee joint, including sartorius, graci-

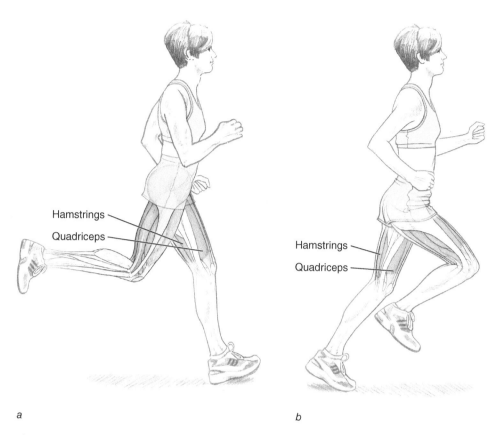

Hamstrings
Quadriceps

Hamstrings
Quadriceps

a   b

Figure 4.6 Muscle activity (a) immediately after heel strike and (b) near the end of the stance phase. At these two points the knee is near full extension, and the hamstring muscles must act as stabilizers.

lis, popliteus, and iliotibial (IT) band (via action of the tensor fasciae latae), serve to minimize transverse plane motions of knee internal and external rotation.

Thus, considering the knee undergoes approximately 40° of sagittal plane flexion, as opposed to 3° of frontal plane and 9° of transverse plane motion, and based on the dominance of the vasti muscles in supporting and controlling the knee joint, adequate strength and function of these muscles is critical for typical knee mechanics. Reduced force output from the vasti muscles because of muscle weakness results in increased knee flexion during the stance phase of gait since these muscles are unable to eccentrically control knee flexion. Arnold et al. (2005) conducted a study utilizing a 3D, muscle-actuated dynamic simulation of gait to understand the relative contributions of hip and knee muscles during normal gait. Overall, the vasti muscles were reported to play a large role in eccentrically controlling knee flexion during stance. Since anterior tibial shear is reduced as the knee flexes, the increase in knee flexion causes a decrease in shear forces and a reduced demand on the hamstring muscles (Osternig et al. 2000; Ferber et al. 2002a; Ferber et al. 2002b; Ferber et al. 2003). On the other hand, reduced hamstring strength, and a concomitant inability to control knee extension at or near heel strike, results in a more flexed knee at heel strike and throughout stance, concomitant reductions in anterior tibial shear, and thus greater demand on the quadriceps muscles to eccentrically control the knee.

 See online video 4.3 for an example of a runner who shows excessive knee flexion.

ANATOMICAL ALIGNMENT

It has been postulated that differences in knee anatomical structure may predispose runners to differences in running mechanics, which over many repetitions may lead to certain injuries. Specifically, a larger Q-angle (figure 4.7) has been reported to be associated with an increase in lateral patellar contact forces (Mizuno et al. 2001). Therefore, an increased Q-angle is thought to lead to a more pronounced genu valgum position during the stance phase of gait and plays a partial role in the etiology of knee-related injuries (DeHaven and Lintner 1986; Messier et al. 1991; Almeida et al. 1999). However, there is very little evidence within the scientific literature regarding the interrelationship between Q-angle and lower-extremity biomechanics.

It has been theorized that Q-angle measures greater than 15° should be considered pathological and be associated with atypical gait mechanics (Caylor et al. 1993; Byl et al. 2000; Heiderscheit et al. 2000). Unfortunately, there is no research data to support this theory. Kernozek and Greer (1993) conducted a study to understand the relationship between Q-angle and rearfoot motion in walking. They conducted a 2D video analysis on 20 women walking on a treadmill and measured static and dynamic Q-angle measures. Overall, the authors reported poor to very poor correlations among the variables and concluded that Q-angle had little to do with predicting or influencing rearfoot motion during gait.

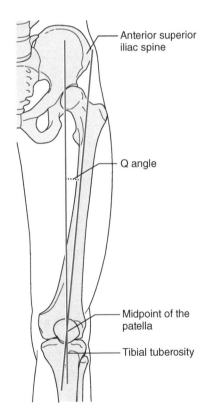

Figure 4.7 Measurement of the Q-angle.

Heiderscheit et al. (1999) assessed the influence of Q-angle on the 3D rearfoot, tibia, and knee joint coupling and coupling variability during gait. Thirty-two subjects had clinical measures of static Q-angle and ran over-ground. Using a unique continuous relative phase (CRP) approach to measure segment couplings to assess between-trial consistency for the stance phase, they reported no differences in CRP variability among subjects with varying Q-angles. In a follow-up study, Heiderscheit et al. (2000) reanalyzed the same data for differences in specific joint angles. Specifically, they hypothesized that an individual with a Q-angle greater than 15° would exhibit increased rearfoot eversion and tibial internal rotation as a result of a greater knee genu valgum angle as compared with those with a Q-angle less than 15°. However, Q-angle measures did not increase the maximum segment or joint angles during running, but the high-Q-angle group demonstrated an increased time to maximum tibial internal rotation. Thus, based on these studies investigating gait biomechanics and the interrelationship to static measures of Q-angle, the conclusion has been that no relationship exists. However, one significant reason for the findings may be the lack of evidence to define a high or low Q-angle.

As previously mentioned, there is no evidence to support the theory that a Q-angle measure greater than 15° is pathological and increases injury risk. In a review article, Livingston (1998) also stated that a high-risk Q-angle measure of 15° to 20° was not based on any scientific literature and was more speculative than evidence based. Subsequently, one study sought to establish a normative range for Q-angle in an asymptomatic population, and adjusted these normative values in accordance with individual-specific mediolateral patellar displacement (Herrington and Nester 2004). Adjusting for patellar displacement is important because an accurate Q-angle measurement depends on a patella centralized within the femoral trochlear groove. If the patella is laterally displaced, the Q-angle measured will be falsely low, and if it is medially displaced, the angle will be falsely high (figure 4.8). These authors reported Q-angle values between 11° and 14° (±5°) for both the left and right knees and for male and female subjects. When correcting for a laterally displaced patella, present in 68 of the 109 subjects tested, a reduction in Q-angle close to 1° was found, but no change was seen when correcting for a medially displaced patella, which was present in 28 subjects.

Moreover, in Livingston's review article (1998), minimum Q-angle values from a variety of peer-reviewed manuscripts for healthy females ranged from 2.5° to 10°, and maximum values ranged from 15° to 26°. As well, while it is commonly assumed that women tend to have larger Q-angles than men, minimum values for healthy males ranged from 0° to 8°, and maximum values ranged from 15° to 27°. Other authors have reported a variety of Q-angle measures ranging from 8° to 14° and 11° to 20° based on measures from 50 men and women, respectively (Horton and Hall 1989), and another study reported ranges of 5° to 16° and 6° to 17° based on measures from 50 men and women, respectively (Livingston and Mandigo 1997). Woodland and Francis (1992) measured the Q-angles of

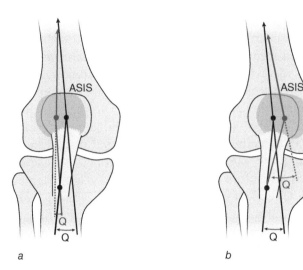

Figure 4.8 *(a)* Medially and *(b)* laterally displaced patella and change in Q-angle.

Based on data from L. Herrington and C. Nester, 2004, "Q-angle undervalued? The relationship between Q-angle and medio-lateral position of the patella," *Clinical Biomechanics* 19(10): 1070-1073.

269 men and 257 women and reported mean values of 13° and 17°, respectively. Thus, when considering Q-angle, values in excess of 15° would fall within normal limits, and the data do not support an across-the-board difference in Q-angle between men and women.

Limited evidence suggests that a very large Q-angle measure (greater than 20°) may increase the risk of injury. Rauh et al. (2007) measured the Q-angle for 393 high school cross-country runners and followed them during a cross-country season to track lower extremity injuries from practices or competitions. They concluded that runners with a Q-angle greater than 20° were at 1.7 times greater risk of injury compared with runners whose Q-angle was between 10° and 15°. Moreover, runners with more than 4° side-to-side difference in Q-angle measures were 1.8 times more likely to sustain an injury than runners with a smaller side-to-side difference. In contrast, another prospective study (Raissi et al. 2009) followed 66 athletes for 17 weeks and reported that Q-angle was not a predictive factor, nor did it increase the relative risk for incurring a running-related injury. However, the measures of Q-angle only ranged between 11° and 13° for both injured and noninjured runners.

In summary, a Q-angle less than 20° should be considered typical based on the aforementioned studies. The long-standing theory of a 15° Q-angle being related to injury is not supported by the literature, and practitioners must take care when attributing a running-related injury solely to a nonmodifiable factor such as Q-angle. Other factors, such as muscle flexibility should also be incorporated into the assessment to better understand atypical mechanical loading to the knee joint.

FLEXIBILITY

While several other muscles and tissues, including the IT band, adductor magnus, and sartorius, cross the knee joint, the paucity of research involving these tissues does not allow us to discuss their potential contributions to typical or atypical knee joint gait mechanics. Previous research has focused primarily on hamstring and quadriceps muscle flexibility in attempts to understand injury etiology.

Flexibility of the hamstring muscles is a critical component to injury prevention. Chumanov et al. (2011) investigated whether the hamstrings are susceptible to injury during the swing phase, when the hamstrings are eccentrically lengthening, or during stance, when knee stabilization and resistance to anterior tibial shear is needed. Using a modeling technique, they measured hamstring lengthening from mid to late swing and shortening under load throughout stance. The authors concluded that the large inertial loads produced from knee extension during the swing phase of gait make the hamstrings most susceptible to injury. Moreover, lateral hamstring (biceps femoris) loading increased significantly with speed and loading was greater during swing than stance. Theoretically, reduced hamstring muscle flexibility and tissue length result in a shortened stride length, increase stride frequency, and reduced knee flexion position at heel strike similar to reduced hamstring muscle strength. The key factor then is to establish the normative range for hamstring tissue flexibility.

Youdas et al. (2005) examined the factors of gender and age over 10-year increments on hamstring muscle length via measurements of passive straight-leg raise and popliteal angle. Overall, females exhibited greater overall hamstring flexibility for both measures (8° greater and 11° greater, respectively) but no differences were measured across age. The mean hamstring muscle length for passive straight-leg raise was 69° (± 7°) for men and 76° (± 10°) for women. When measuring hamstring flexibility via popliteal angle, the authors reported values of 141° (± 8°) for men and 152° (± 11°) for women. Using these hamstring flexibility values, practitioners and runners can determine if they are at risk for atypical knee joint loads or atypical running biomechanics.

An interesting study by Silder et al. (2010) investigated whether residual scar tissue at the hamstring musculotendon junction after a previous injury would influence strength, neuromotor activation patterns, and joint kinematics. While magnetic resonance (MR) imaging revealed significantly enlarged proximal biceps femoris tendon volume for the injured hamstring muscle, no significant between-limb differences were found for any other variables. The authors concluded that previous hamstring injuries and residual scar tissue did not negatively influence function or gait mechanics. However, it is unknown whether the hamstring muscles exhibited reduced flexibility concomitant with the enlarged tendon volume.

Few investigations have been conducted to evaluate quadriceps muscle flexibility as a risk factor for injury. A review article from van der Worp et al. (2011) suggested only poor to moderate evidence for nine factors related to patellar tendinopathy, including reduced quadriceps flexibility. However, the authors stressed a clear need for high-quality studies. Considering the knee undergoes approximately 40° of knee flexion during the stance phase of gait, and the vasti muscles produce the majority of support to the knee joint, adequate flexibility is critical to allow for normal range of knee motion. If the vasti muscles are inflexible, there would be a reduced amount of knee flexion during stance in contrast to the changes due to reduced vasti strength. Unfortunately, even fewer studies have established normative ranges for quadriceps muscle flexibility, but Harvey (1998) measured quadriceps flexibility via knee flexion angle during the Thomas test and reported a mean angle of 53°.

 See online video 4.4 for an example of a runner who shows reduced knee flexion.

In summary, while muscle flexibility has been shown to play a minor role in injury etiology and prevention as the primary causative factor, there is still some research needed to help identify when the degrees of hamstring and quadriceps muscle flexibility are within normal limits and not a factor in injury prevention and rehabilitation. Considering that limited hamstring flexibility has been linked to a shortened stride length, optimal flexibility is important from a running performance standpoint.

SUMMARY

As we move up the kinematic chain we start to see that the relative coupling and joint motions between the foot, tibia, and femur begin to get complicated. However, by maintaining our process for determining the interrelationships among biomechanical, strength, flexibility, and anatomical alignment, we can sort through the data and begin to understand our patients' overall gait mechanics. Certainly the knee is most predisposed to running-related injuries and as we continue up the kinematic chain and begin to discuss hip biomechanics in chapter 5, we'll develop both a distal-to-proximal and a proximal-to-distal method of gait analysis.

Assessing Hip Mechanics

The final joint to consider as we move up the kinematic chain is the hip joint. Over the past 15 years, several research studies have focused on the hip as a key determinant in injury prediction and optimal rehabilitation. As discussed for the ankle and knee joints, we focus first on biomechanics observed during gait and then discuss the interrelationships among strength, anatomical alignment, and muscle flexibility.

BIOMECHANICS

For the first half of stance, while the knee joint undergoes flexion, internal rotation, and abduction, the hip functions in a similar manner (figures 5.1-5.3). Specifically, at heel strike the hip is approximately 30° flexed and remains in this position for about the first 30% to 40% of stance. Thus, it is flexion at the knee joint that primarily brings the center of mass downward during this period of time. For the remaining 60% to 70% of stance, the hip undergoes extension and is nearly fully extended at toe-off (figure 5.1).

Throughout the beginning of stance, the hip also adducts and internally rotates (figure 5.2). However, since the swing leg is bringing the pelvis anteriorly and the transverse plane motion of the pelvis is opposite (external rotation) to the femur, there is little internal rotation (2°-3°) at the hip joint as compared with the 9° rotation at the knee joint. Thus, overall transverse plane motion at the hip is primarily composed of external rotation, which begins at approximately 20% of stance. At toe-off the hip is in an externally rotated position as a result of pelvic transverse plane motion (figure 5.3). For the second half of stance, the hip abducts in a manner similar to the knee but greater in overall magnitude. Thus, just as the coupling and timing relationship between the knee and rearfoot was asynchronous, the timing between the hip and knee joints is asynchronous as well.

Several authors have also reported these asynchronous patterns and out-of-phase relationships during the stance phase of gait for hip internal rotation and tibial internal rotation (Hamill et al. 1999; Dierks and Davis 2007). Unlike the relationship between rearfoot eversion and tibial internal rotation, both the

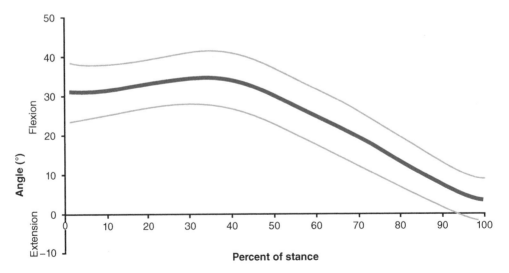

Figure 5.1 Biomechanical motion of hip sagittal plane motion during the stance phase of running gait. A stance of 0% indicates heel strike, and a stance of 100% indicates toe-off.

Note: Blue line = mean; gray lines = ± 1 SD.

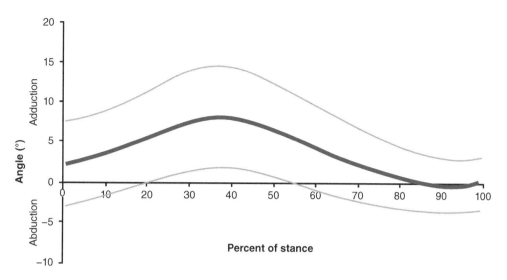

Figure 5.2 Biomechanical motion of hip frontal plane motion during the stance phase of running gait. 0% of stance indicates heel strike, and 100% of stance indicates toe-off.
Note: Blue line = mean; gray lines = ± 1 SD.

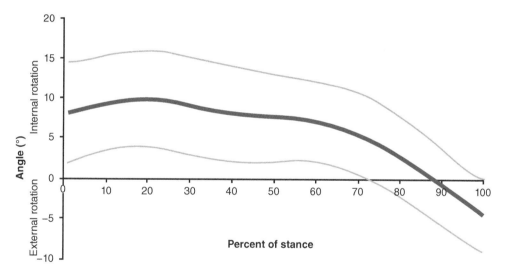

Figure 5.3 Biomechanical motion of hip transverse plane motion during the stance phase of running gait. 0% of stance indicates heel strike and 100% of stance indicates toe-off.
Note: Blue line = mean; gray lines = ± 1 SD.

hip's and knee's transverse plane relationships remain uncoupled throughout stance, and studies have reported this relationship to be largely nonsystematic across subjects. These results are surprising because these motions are thought to occur synchronously. It has been theorized that the out-of-phase nature of these relationships may be a function of the velocities of these motions, with the tibia and knee rotating more quickly than the hip. With this lack of movement synchrony and timing, it is no surprise that the knee joint is most susceptible to injury. There is a large amount of coupling variability between the knee and ankle joints, and there is relatively no synchronous coupling between the knee and hip joints. Considering that the tibia and knee rotate much more quickly and to a larger degree than the hip joint, the knee is much more susceptible to injury even under typical biomechanical circumstances.

 See online videos 5.1a and b for posterior and anterior views of typical hip mechanics during running.

STRENGTH

As previously mentioned, from foot flat to 20% of stance, the vasti muscles along with the gluteus maximus and medius produce the majority of support and prevent the knee and hip from collapsing against the downward pull of gravity and during knee flexion. Since the hip remains in approximately 30° of flexion for this period of time, the gluteal muscles are contracting isometrically to maintain this static hip flexion position (figure 5.4a). During midstance and with significant passive resistance from noncontractile tissues such as the hip joint capsule and ligaments, the gluteus medius and minimus provide nearly all of the support to accelerate the center of mass upward as the hip joint begins to extend. Thus, gluteus maximus begins to contract concentrically, along with assistance from the hamstring muscles, to produce the overall hip extension motion (figure

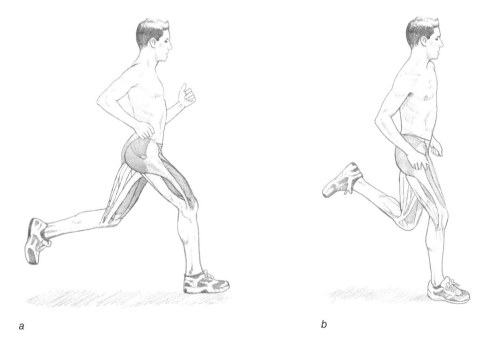

a   b

Figure 5.4 Gluteal and hamstring activity during (a) the early stance phase and (b) midstance.

5.4*b*) (Anderson and Pandy 2003; Pandy and Andriacchi 2010). In fact, based on per unit of force, the gluteus maximus has greater potential compared with the vasti muscles to control knee flexion, which is discussed later in this chapter.

With respect to frontal plane motion, Pandy et al. (2010) reported that the body's center of mass accelerates outward and downward during the first half of stance. The vasti muscles and the gluteus maximus serve to support the downward acceleration and prevent collapse. Interestingly, only the gluteus medius muscle functions to accelerate the body medially (inward) and thus maintains overall mediolateral balance (figure 5.5). Based on these data, several authors have hypothesized that a primary contributing factor to running-related injuries is weakness of the gluteus medius musculature and the subsequent alterations in frontal plane hip and knee motion (Ireland et al. 2003; Mascal et al. 2003; Cichanowski et al. 2007; Robinson and Nee 2007; Bolgla et al. 2008; Dierks et al. 2008; Willson and Davis 2008).

The gluteus medius has been theorized to eccentrically control hip adduction, and thus knee genu valgum angle, during the stance phase of gait (Ferber et al. 2003; Ireland et al. 2003; Mascal et al. 2003; Powers 2003; Cichanowski et al. 2007; Robinson and Nee 2007; Bolgla et al. 2008; Dierks et al. 2008; Willson and Davis 2008). Unfortunately, few studies have examined the relationship between gluteus medius muscle strength and hip and knee mechanics. Bolgla et al. (2008) measured gluteus medius strength and knee and hip kinematics and reported that subjects with patellofemoral pain syndrome (PFPS) exhibited reduced muscle force output but no differences in knee genu valgum angle during a stair descent compared with controls.

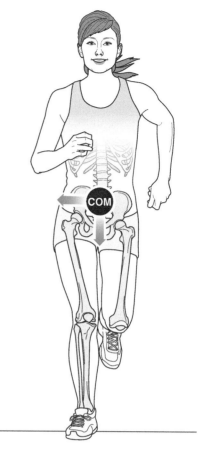

Figure 5.5 During the first half of stance, the body's center of mass is accelerating outward and downward, which requires the hip muscles to act as stabilizers to maintain balance.

 See online videos 5.2*a* to *c* for an example of a runner with excessive hip adduction and pelvic drop.

Similarly, Dierks et al. (2008) measured reduced gluteus medius isometric force output for subjects with PFPS and control subjects after an exhaustive run. However, in contrast to Bolgla et al. (2008), the PFPS patients in this fatigue study exhibited an increase in peak hip adduction over the course of the run compared to the healthy runners. These data suggest that reduced force output from the gluteus medius will result in an increased hip adduction angle and thus a greater knee genu valgum (abduction) angle during gait. However, Snyder et al. (2009) reported that after a 6-week hip strengthening protocol, healthy female runners exhibited a 13% gain in abductor strength, but the hip adduction angle during running increased by 1.4°, contrary to their hypotheses and the afore-mentioned studies. So it is unclear exactly how fatigue or reduced force output from this muscle group can influence hip and knee biomechanics during gait.

We sought to test the hypothesis of whether improvements in muscle strength would lead to a reduced peak knee genu valgum angle for runners with PFPS. We conducted an experiment involving 15 runners with PFPS and 10 healthy runners (Ferber, Kendall, et al. 2011). All subjects were involved in a 3-week hip abductor muscle-strengthening protocol composed of two exercises. We found that over a 3-week protocol, the level of pain experienced by the PFPS patients decreased on average 40% and there was a 33% improvement in strength, but no changes in the peak knee abduction angle occurred. However, we took a novel approach to understanding potential changes in gait mechanics and measured the stride-to-stride kinematic pattern. We found a more consistent frontal plane knee movement pattern concomitant with the gains in strength. We theorized that by providing the knee with a more consistent stride-to-stride movement pattern, a more optimal environment is established to allow for tissue healing and pain resolution. We also repeated this study with another group of 20 PFPS runners (Ferber, Bolga, et al. 2011), using the same rehabilitation exercises used by Snyder et al. (2009). Similar to our first study, we found that baseline movement variability was higher for the PFPS involved knee and hip joints compared to controls. Also contrary to the hypotheses, the PFPS affected leg demonstrated reduced knee and hip movement variability after a 6-week strengthening inter-vention. We concluded that stride-to-stride knee joint variability may be a better indicator of atypical gait patterns compared with peak angles, and it highlighted the importance of understanding the interrelationship between hip abductor muscle strength and biomechanical assessment.

ANATOMICAL ALIGNMENT

We do not measure aspects of hip or pelvis anatomical structure within our clinical and biomechanical assessment. The primary reason for this decision is that there are very few scientific investigations related to the reliability or validity of hip and pelvic alignment measures. However, we do measure leg length discrepancy (LLD) based on the scientific literature and its relationship to biomechanics and joint injury.

Leg length discrepancy is assessed with subjects positioned supine after the **Weber-Barstow maneuver**, (figure 5.6) is used to set the pelvis (McGee 2007). See figure 5.6. Overall, it is accepted that a LLD is present when more than a

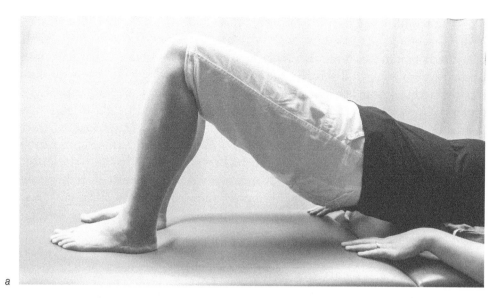

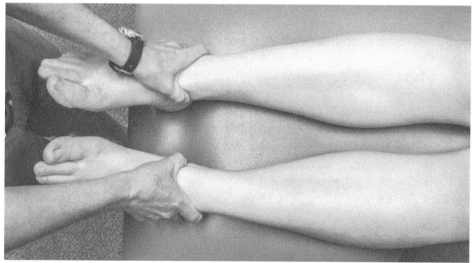

Figure 5.6 *(a)* the Weber-Barstow maneuver and *(b)* assessment of leg length discrepancy.

2 cm side-to-side difference is radiographically confirmed (Perttunen et al. 2004). However, this discrepancy has not been well defined, and the literature does not support this value through comprehensive research studies. We conducted a study to provide a comprehensive database from a large population of runners with selected anatomical alignment measures commonly associated with running injuries (Kendall et al. 2008). We measured 221consecutive patients that presented to the clinic for various musculoskeletal running injuries. The average LLD was 0.45 cm (± 0.87 cm), and only 3.17% of patients exhibited a LLD greater than 1.5 cm. Thus, we concluded that LLD, unless radiographically confirmed, is rare within an active, injured population.

LLD may influence overall gait mechanics. Unfortunately, very few studies have been conducted to confirm or refute this supposition. Perttunen et al. (2004) measured plantar pressures and 2D ground reaction forces on 25 patients with confirmed limb length discrepancy of more than 2 cm. Overall, these authors reported reduced stance time in the short leg and greater peak plantar pressure under the first ray in the long leg. They concluded that loading of the long limb is greater and the forefoot of the long limb experiences greater loading than the short limb. Finally, White et al. (2004) also reported that the shorter limb sustains a greater proportion of load and loading rates compared with the longer limb. However, some anatomic LLDs investigated in this study were between 1-1.5 cm, which are within normal limits for the vast majority of runners, and therefore may not be clinically relevant.

FLEXIBILITY

The key flexibility measures for the hip are the internal rotation range of motion and tissue flexibility of the rectus femoris, iliopsoas, and iliotibial (IT) band. Biomechanically, the hip internally rotates during early stance and therefore requires sufficient **hip rotation** range of motion to allow this motion to occur. If the hip cannot adequately internally rotate, increased torsional stress is created within the hip, knee, and ankle joints. To minimize this torsional stress, the hip could return to an externally rotated position, but the relative external rotation of the pelvis, as the swing leg is moving forward and driving the pelvis into an externally rotated position, prevents the unloading, or external rotation, of the hip joint. Thus, sufficient hip internal range of motion flexibility is critical for the reduction in torsional stress.

The rationale behind increased torsional stress being a predictor of injury was first proposed by Holden and Cavanagh (1991). These authors calculated the free moment, the rotational force the foot applies to the ground during the stance phase of gait. Specifically, they reported that the free moment was greatest during the first half of stance and acted to resist foot abduction, a component of overall foot pronation. Additionally, they reported that with greater amounts of rearfoot eversion, the free moment increased. In chapter 6 we discuss the free moment in greater detail.

Unfortunately, few studies have investigated the role of hip rotator strengthening for the treatment of musculoskeletal injuries, and none have determined whether improvements in rotator range of motion influences torsional forces. However, Cibulka and Threlkeld-Watkins (2005) reported a case study involving a 15-year-old who had been experiencing anterior right knee pain for 8 months. Clinical investigation revealed reduced internal rotation flexibility of the right hip and external rotator strength compared to the left, and a rehabilitation program was designed to improve these factors. After 6 visits, within 14 days, the patient's side-to-side asymmetry was negligible, and the pain was gone. While this study is the only one involving a focused, hip rotator rehabilitation program, and the limitations of being a case study are evident, it does provide evidence of the role of improved rotator flexibility for the treatment of knee pain.

On the other hand, increased or excessive hip internal rotation range of motion must be matched with appropriate rotator muscle strength. If the excessive hip rotation range of motion is measured, increased mechanical internal rotation can occur during the stance phase of gait, resulting in increased torsional stress at the hip and especially knee joint. Souza and Powers (2009) reported that 19 female athletes with PFPS exhibited significantly greater than average hip internal rotation range of motion and reduced isotonic hip muscle strength in 8 of 10 hip strength measurements as compared with controls. The authors suggested that excessive internal rotation range of motion must be matched with improvements in overall hip muscle strength to minimize atypical biomechanical motion.

With respect to rectus femoris and IT band flexibility testing, the special tests used by clinicians for assessing these tissues are highly subjective and involve either a positive or negative assessment, making it difficult to apply within evidence-based medicine. While some studies have used either goniometers or inclinometers to quantify the modified Thomas test or Obers test, very few have established normative values.

For rectus femoris and iliopsoas, Corkery et al. (2007) reported on values for various muscle lengths for 72 college-age students using a goniometer. They reported on the modified Thomas test for iliopsoas and the Thomas test for rectus femoris. The modified Thomas test methodology Corkery used involved having the subject lie supine with the body completely on a table that prevented the thigh from dropping below the table (figure 5.7), and thus an average angle of

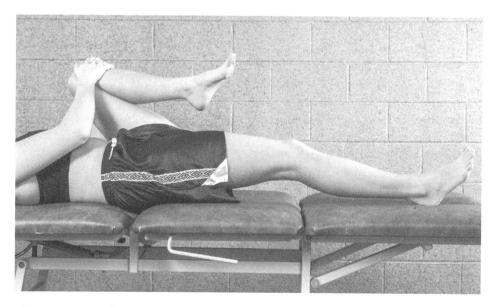

Figure 5.7   Modified Thomas test.

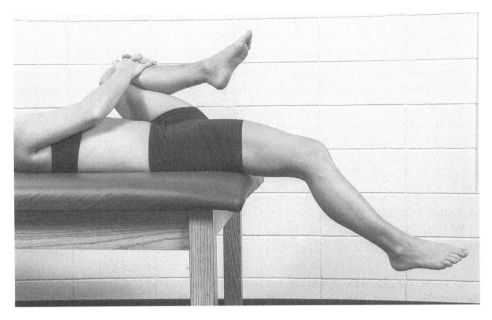

Figure 5.8 Thomas test.

© Human Kinetics

2.3° (± 1.8°) above the horizontal was reported for the iliopsoas. The Thomas test involved sitting on the edge of the table and allowing the thigh to drop (figure 5.8). They reported an average angle of 52.8° (± 10.5°) for the rectus femoris. Harvey (1998) assessed the flexibility of the iliopsoas using a goniometer for 117 elite athletes and allowed the thigh to drop below the horizontal. They reported an average angle of 11.91° below the horizontal.

We conducted a study (Ferber et al. 2010) to compare the subjective evaluation of iliopsoas flexibility to the instrumented measurement of a digital inclinometer in the hopes of establishing normative values and providing a critical criterion. Three hundred recreational athletes were classified subjectively as either positive or negative for IT band and iliopsoas tightness using the Ober's and Thomas test, respectively. A digital inclinometer measured thigh position relative to the horizontal to the nearest tenth of a degree. For iliopsoas flexibility, the average inclinometer angle was consistent with Harvey (1998) and was -10.60 ± 9.61°. Interestingly, 208 limbs were subjectively assessed as positive (0.34 ± 7.00°) and 392 limbs were assessed as negative (-15.51 ± 5.82°) and the between-clinician agreement was 95.0%. Thus, a Thomas test measuring less than 10° below the horizontal should be considered atypical and related to reduced iliopsoas tissue flexibility. A modified Thomas test greater than 2.3° above the horizontal should be considered atypical and related to reduced rectus femoris tissue flexibility.

It has been hypothesized that reduced iliopsoas tissue flexibility would result in reduced peak hip extension, stride length, and gait speed during gait (Watt et al. 2011). A study by Kerrigan et al. (2003) performed a double-blinded, randomized, controlled trial wherein 96 healthy elderly individuals were allocated into a treatment and control group. The treatment group received a one-time instruction in hip flexor stretching, and the control group received a one-time instruction in shoulder abductor stretching. After a 1.6° (± 3.0°) improvement in hip flexor flexibility, the treatment group demonstrated a 2°, but statistically nonsignificant, increase in peak hip extension during walking. Interestingly, a significant improvement in peak ankle plantar flexion angle was measured and attributed to improvements in hip flexor contracture rather than changes at the ankle. Watt et al. (2011) conducted another double-blinded, randomized, controlled trial for 74 frail older adults over a 10-week program of twice-daily hip flexor stretching. Similar to Kerrigan et al. (2003) the authors reported significant improvements in passive iliopsoas flexibility and significant increases in gait velocity and stride length during walking, but there were no significant changes in peak hip extension. Based on these intervention studies, improvements in hip flexor flexibility do not seem to coincide with significant improvements in peak hip extension. Future studies that involve a more active population and take into consideration trunk mechanics and flexibility of other muscles are necessary.

Very few studies have been conducted to establish a normative range for IT band tissue flexibility using the Obers test (figure 5.9). In the aforementioned study (Ferber et al. 2010) we also measured the modified Obers test using a digital inclinometer to establish IT band flexibility. We reported an average angle of –24.59° for all 300 participants regardless of whether they were subjectively deemed to exhibit a positive or negative position. Of the 600 limbs of interest, 168 were subjectively assessed as positive while 432 were assessed as negative. The critical criterion for the Obers test was –23.16°. Hudson and Darthuy (2009) also measured IT band tightness in a group of 12 control subjects and 12 subjects with PFPS using a bubble inclinometer. The authors reported a range of –20.3° to –21.4° for the controls and –14.9° to –17.3° for the PFPS group, which are similar to the results of our study. Thus, an Obers test measuring less than 20° below the horizontal should be considered atypical and related to reduced IT band tissue flexibility.

It has been theorized that the primary functions of the IT band are to serve as a lateral hip and knee stabilizer and to resist hip adduction and knee internal rotation (Fredericson et al. 2000). The iliotibial band originates from the fibers of the gluteus maximus, gluteus medius, and tensor fasciae latae muscles and attaches proximal to the knee joint into the lateral femoral condyle and distal to the knee joint into the intercondylar tubercle of the tibia (Birnbaum et al. 2004). As a result of the femoral and tibial attachments, it is possible that abnormal hip as well as foot mechanics, which both influence the knee, could play a role in the development of IT band syndrome or IT band tightness.

Because the iliotibial band attaches to the lateral condyle of the tibia, it is postulated that excessive rearfoot eversion resulting in greater tibial internal rotation could increase the strain in the iliotibial band. Miller et al. (2007) reported that at the end of an exhaustive run, runners with IT band syndrome

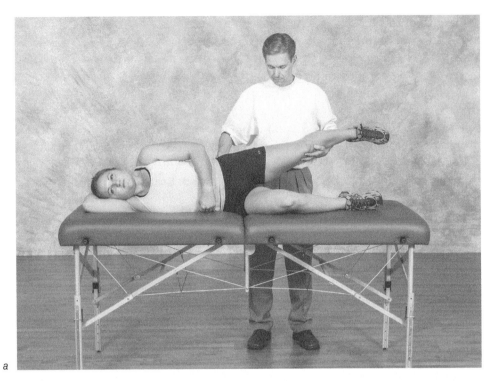

a

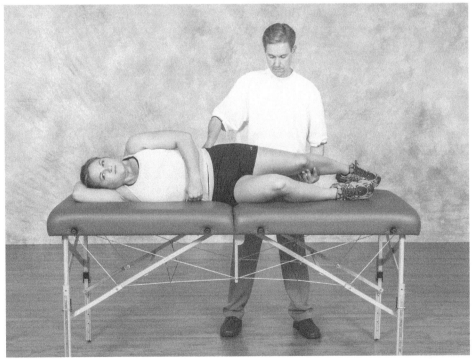

b

Figure 5.9 Obers test *(a)* start position and *(b)* lowering the leg to test IT band flexibility.

© Human Kinetics

demonstrated a greater rearfoot inversion angle at heel strike compared with controls, which the researchers hypothesized contributed to a greater peak knee and tibial internal rotation velocity and thus increased torsional strain to the IT band. In contrast, Messier et al. (1995) reported that runners with a history of IT band syndrome exhibited no difference in rearfoot mechanics compared with healthy runners. Moreover, since the gluteus medius muscle is the primary abductor of the hip joint, weakness of this muscle may lead to an increased hip adduction angle, thereby potentially increasing the strain on the IT band. Fredericson et al. (2000) reported that runners with IT band syndrome had significantly reduced hip abductor muscle strength in the affected limb compared with the unaffected limb, as well as compared with healthy controls. However, very few studies have investigated whether atypical hip mechanics may play a role in the etiology of ITBS.

A prospective study by Noehren et al. (2007) and a retrospective study by Ferber et al. 2010 examined proximal (hip), distal (rearfoot), as well as local (knee) mechanics in the development of IT band syndrome. For both studies, the IT band syndrome group exhibited significantly greater peak knee internal rotation angle and peak hip adduction angle compared to the healthy runners, but no significant differences in peak rearfoot eversion angle or peak knee flexion angle were observed between groups. The common results between the prospective study and the retrospective study provide strong evidence related to atypical running mechanics and the etiology of ITBS.

SUMMARY

We have now journeyed up the kinematic chain and thoroughly discussed the biomechanical gait patterns of the ankle, knee, and hip joints. The complexity of the interrelationships between strength, flexibility, and anatomical alignment make a gait assessment a task best approached in a systematic manner. In chapter 6 we present case studies to help give context to typical and atypical biomechanical patterns and how these patterns are related to the other three factors.

Proximal to Distal Relationships: Case Studies

Now that many aspects of lower extremity biomechanics, strength, flexibility, and anatomical alignment factors have been discussed, we tie together these concepts through three case studies that demonstrate the interrelationship of ankle, knee, and hip biomechanics as they relate to specific injuries. We start with a discussion of overall torsional forces through a related case study, then address issues and cases related to frontal plane movement.

TORSIONAL FORCES

Our first case study discusses a novel approach to understanding and identifying increased torsional forces through measures and visual observations of a runner's **heel whip**. Torsional forces are commonly experienced during running, and increased torsional forces are hypothesized to be related to musculoskeletal injury etiology. The biomechanical measure of torsional force during the stance phase of gait is called the *free moment*. The free moment is the torque about a vertical axis due to friction between the foot and the ground during stance (Holden and Cavanagh 1991). It is the resistance to toeing out during the stance phase of gait when the foot is fixed to the ground as a result of high frictional shoe–ground forces (figure 6.1). While the free moment has been linked to the amount of foot pronation, its relationship to other factors such as muscular strength, flexibility, and anatomical alignment has not been investigated. However, certain assumptions can be drawn based on the current literature.

It has been speculated that a higher free moment is likely related to a higher amount of torque experienced within the lower extremity. Milner et al. (2004) reported that a higher free moment was measured in 13 runners with a history of tibial stress fractures compared with runners with no previous lower-extremity bony injuries. In a follow-up study, these same authors reported that the peak free moment had a significant predictive relationship for runners with a history of tibial stress fractures (Milner et al. 2006). Other authors have also investigated the free moment and reported that individuals who ambulate with a more externally rotated foot position exhibit a greater peak free moment compared with a more internally rotated foot alignment (Almosnino et al. 2009). A more externally rotated foot may be the result of reduced hip internal rotation range of motion or hip external rotator strength (as discussed in chapter 5) or other nonmodifiable factors such as increased tibial torsion or femoral anteversion.

The free moment can only be measured using a force plate during overground running or via an instrumented treadmill. Previous research has shown that the free moment increases significantly with increases in foot pronation since the free moment is greatest in magnitude during the first half of stance as it acts in a direction resisting foot abduction, which is a component of pronation (Holden and Cavanagh 1991). Thus, if increased foot pronation is measured or observed, then increased torsional forces are experienced

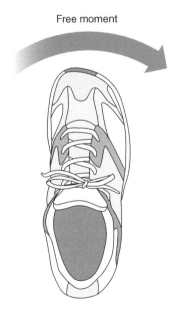

Free moment

Figure 6.1 The free moment during the stance phase of gait, showing the resistance to toeing out when the foot is fixed to the ground.

within the lower extremity. The fact that, as a part of typical biomechanical gait patterns, the tibia internally rotates while the talus adducts (discussed in chapter 2) further supports the link between increased foot pronation and increased torsional stress (figures 2.2-2.4). Since the free moment is the resistance to toeing out, and because foot pronation is mechanically coupled with tibial and femoral internal rotation, increased torsional forces are assumed to occur while the foot is in contact with the ground. Since toe-off is the first opportunity for the lower extremity to return to an externally rotated position, the heel whips medially as the leg rotates outward, back to a resting position, and is an indicator of the torsional stress that has built up in the lower extremity (figure 6.2).

▶ **See online video 6.1 for an example of a runner showing a medial heel whip.**

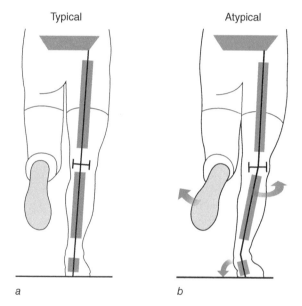

Figure 6.2 *(a)* Non-heel-whip position for the left foot compared with *(b)* an outwardly rotating left foot and the subsequent heel whip.

Case Study: Tibialis Posterior Tendinopathy

The first case study is a runner presenting with bilateral tibialis posterior tendinopathy (TPT) with greater right-side symptoms and pain.

 See online videos 6.2a and b. The runner in these clips is experiencing tibialis posterior tendinopathy as described in this case study.

INJURY HISTORY

The tendinopathy began on the right side close to 6 months ago, and within the past 2 months the left tendinopathy began. The runner received direct local treatment consisting of ultrasound, ice, and gastrocnemius and soleus stretching. In addition, the runner completed isolated tibialis posterior strengthening exercises as well as a calf-raise program progressing up to single-leg calf raises for 3 sets of 20 repetitions over 4 weeks. Finally, 2 months ago, she received a pair of custom-made orthotics to help reduce the dynamic strain to the tibialis posterior by supporting the medial longitudinal arch. The runner also reduced her mileage, stopped running altogether for 3 weeks at a time on two separate occasions, and changed her running shoes twice. While the pain and symptoms were reduced for short periods of time over the past 6 months, the tendinopathy remains recalcitrant and unresolved. Nerve entrapment has begun to present during every run as a result of tarsal tunnel syndrome and entrapment of the tibial nerve because of tendon enlargement and swelling of the tibialis posterior tendon. Our job is to determine the root cause of the injury through consideration of alignment, strength, flexibility, and biomechanics.

Injury History Summary
Conditions
- Tibialis posterior tendinopathy
- Tarsal tunnel syndrome and entrapment of the tibial nerve

Duration
6 months on R, 2 months on L

Symptoms
Pain: R > L

Signs
Tibialis posterior tendon swelling

Previous Treatments
- Ultrasound
- Ice
- Gastrocnemius and soleus stretching
- Isolated tibialis posterior strengthening exercises
- Calf-raise program progressing up to single-leg calf raises

- Custom-made orthotics
- Reduced mileage and stopped running for 3 weeks at a time on two separate occasions
- Changed running shoes two times

ASSESSMENT

All foot and arch anatomical measures are in the high to excessive range except for Q-angle and leg-length discrepancy (figure 6.3). The increased arch height index (a more pes cavus alignment and a stiffer arch), increased standing rearfoot eversion posture, and forefoot varus orientation must be accompanied by sufficient ankle invertor strength to prevent excessive foot pronation and thus tibial internal rotation. Inspection of figure 6.4 shows that this patient exhibits adequate ankle stabilizer strength, and figure 6.5 shows that she exhibits typical rearfoot eversion, time to peak rearfoot eversion, and eversion velocity. Thus, we conclude that the ankle stabilizers are adequately controlling the foot during the stance phase of running. However, a significant amount of tibial internal rotation is measured during midstance suggesting increased torsional forces are experienced at the ankle and knee irrespective of the typical foot pronation biomechanics. In other words, the increased torsional stress is not a result of atypical foot mechanics but rather a more proximal problem.

Inspection of figure 6.6 shows that the knee behaves in a typical biomechanical manner such that the typical knee genu valgum and knee internal

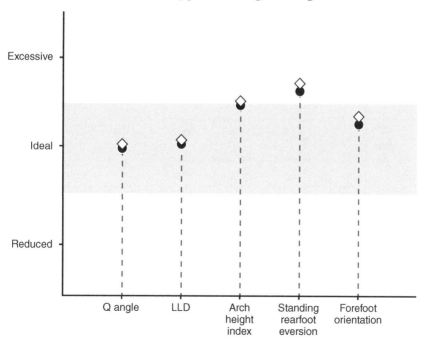

Figure 6.3 Alignment measures.

Note: Diamond = right limb; circle = left limb.

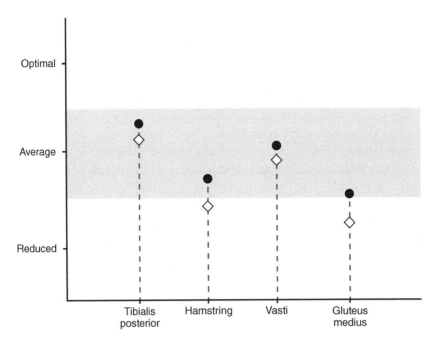

Figure 6.4 Strength measures.
Note: Diamond = right limb; circle = left limb.

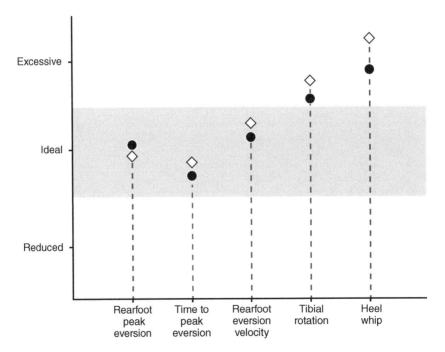

Figure 6.5 Foot biomechanical measures.
Note: Diamond = right limb; circle = left limb.

rotation (distal femur rotation on the tibia) are measured. This is not unexpected considering the typical Q-angle measurement. However, increased hip internal rotation is measured, suggesting that the greater tibial internal rotation is a function of the hip rotating excessively inward. If knee rotation is within normal limits, then one must conclude that both the tibia and femur are rotating inward to the same (greater) degree. The question is why is there excessive hip rotation?

Inspection of figure 6.7 shows that the hip rotator flexibility measures are within normal limits. Thus, the excessive biomechanical hip rotation cannot be attributed to excessive passive hip rotation range of motion. However, figure 6.4 shows low to reduced gluteus medius and hamstring muscle strength. Thus, we conclude that the reduced muscle strength is the primary cause for the increased femoral and tibial rotation (and associated increased hip adduction) and consequently increased tibial rotation biomechanics. The typical foot mechanics measured suggest that the posterior tibial tendinopathy is not the result of atypical foot mechanics, rather it is the increased torsional stress at the ankle joint. Furthermore, the increased medial heel whip, observed in figure 6.3 and in the video of the runner, suggest that while the foot is on the ground, the runner experiences an increased peak free moment. These data suggest that the tibialis posterior must compensate for the lack of hamstring and gluteus medius muscle strength, and thus it undergoes excessive strain to minimize the increased torsional stress at the ankle.

Assessment Summary

Anatomical
- Excessive arch height index
- Excessive standing rearfoot eversion
- Forefoot varus

Strength
- Reduced hamstring strength
- Reduced gluteus medius strength

Foot Biomechanics
- Normal rearfoot peak eversion, time to peak eversion, and eversion velocity
- Increased peak tibial internal rotation
- Excessive heel whip

Knee and Hip Biomechanics
- Excessive peak hip internal rotation
- Increased peak pelvic drop

Flexibility
Normal hip rotator flexibility

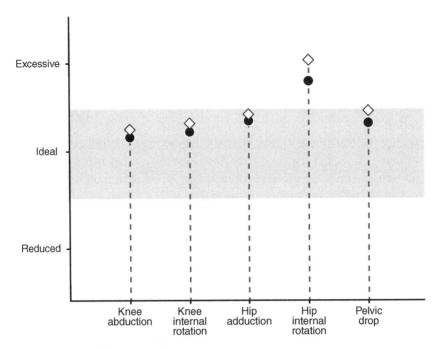

Figure 6.6 Knee and hip biomechanical measures.
Note: Diamond = right limb; circle = left limb.

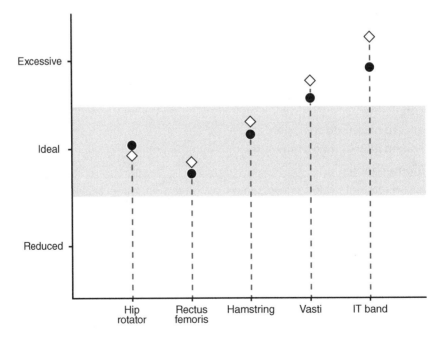

Figure 6.7 Flexibility measures.
Note: Diamond = right limb; circle = left limb.

PRIMARY TREATMENT

Primary treatment for this patient focuses on hamstring and gluteus medius muscle strengthening to reduce the torsional stress experienced at the ankle. Considering that the foot exhibits typical biomechanics, we would recommend that the custom-made orthotics be discontinued and that this patient runs in a neutral or light stability shoe. However, considering the high arch height index measure (a more rigid midfoot) and high to excessive measures of standing rearfoot valgus and forefoot orientation, a neutral foot bed, or over-the-counter orthotic device could be considered. Considering that all flexibility measures are within normal limits, muscle stretching is not a critical component of rehabilitation but could be continued to ensure that scar tissue or adhesions that developed over the past 6 months do not inhibit rehabilitation progress. Local treatment to minimize swelling and adhesion formation could continue but should not be the focus of the rehabilitation plan.

Focus of Treatment
- Strengthen gluteus medius
- Strengthen hamstrings
- Use a neutral or light stability shoe
- Consider arch support

FRONTAL PLANE MECHANICS

Secondary plane forces are considered to be the root cause of most musculoskeletal injuries (McClay and Manal 1999). In this section, we discuss excessive motion and forces along the frontal plane. Specifically, we detail the interrelationship between rearfoot eversion, knee abduction or genu valgum, hip adduction, and pelvic drop during gait. Related to these mechanical factors, the role of frontal plane muscular strength, flexibility of associated tissues, and anatomical alignment are discussed in the context of two case studies.

Case Study: Medial Tibial Stress Syndrome

This case study focuses on a runner presenting with bilateral medial tibial stress syndrome (MTSS or shin splints) with pain and tenderness along the medial tibia.

 See online videos 6.3a to e for footage of a runner experiencing medial tibial stress syndrome as described in this case study.

INJURY HISTORY

The symptoms have increased dramatically over the last month as a result of increased mileage in preparation for an upcoming half marathon. However, during almost every run for the past 12 months, there has been some pain and discomfort at the beginning of each run, subsequent reductions in pain as the run continues, and inevitable pain after the run, which continues until the next day. Over the past 4 months, the patient has switched to motion control shoes; worn gel inserts in those shoes; had direct treatment to the medial aspect of the tibia, including ultrasound, intra-muscular stimulation, and stretching; and reduced her mileage at times to minimize the pain. Our job now is to determine the root cause of the injury by considering alignment, strength, flexibility, and biomechanics.

Injury History Summary
Condition
    Bilateral medial tibial stress syndrome (shin splints)
Duration
    Pain and discomfort for the past 12 months, with a dramatic increase in symptoms over the past month
Symptoms
    Pain: R / L
Signs
    Pain and tenderness along the medial border of the distal 1/3 of the tibia
Previous Treatments
- Switched to motion control shoes
- Gel inserts in shoes
- Ultrasound
- Intramuscular stimulation
- Stretching
- Reduced running mileage

ASSESSMENT

All foot and arch anatomical alignment measures are within normal limits or less than typically measured (figure 6.8). In fact, the patient exhibits a rearfoot

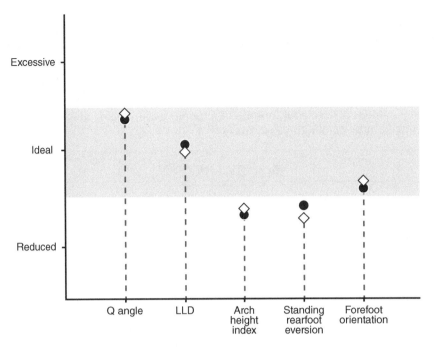

Figure 6.8 Alignment measures.

Note: Diamond = right limb; circle = left limb.

varus standing posture and has a low arch height index, suggesting that we would expect to measure typical or even reduced rearfoot eversion during gait. Based on the information from chapter 3 regarding methods to choose correct footwear, a motion control shoe is not an ideal choice. The slightly high but still within normal limits Q-angle measure may result in excessive hip or knee frontal plane mechanics if sufficient muscle strength is not present. Inspection of figure 6.9 demonstrates that the subject exhibits reduced frontal plane muscle stabilization in terms of the tibialis posterior and gluteus medius musculature.

Figure 6.10 demonstrates excessive and prolonged time to peak rearfoot eversion. We would not necessarily expect excessive rearfoot eversion considering the standing rearfoot varus foot posture and must therefore assume that proximal factors, such as excessive knee abduction (genu valgum), play a role. This hypothesis is reinforced considering that excessive tibial internal rotation is not measured. Remember, tibial internal rotation and rearfoot eversion are coupled motions. If excessive rearfoot eversion is not coupled with excessive tibial internal rotation, the rearfoot is being induced into an excessive eversion position as a result of increased knee abduction (genu valgum) or hip adduction. The prolonged time to peak rearfoot eversion and high eversion velocity is the direct result of reduced tibialis posterior muscle strength and the inability to control rearfoot eversion during the first half of stance and bring the rearfoot into an inverted position during the last half of stance.

Inspection of figure 6.11 shows excessive knee abduction, hip adduction, and contralateral pelvic-drop gait mechanics that are the direct result of reduced

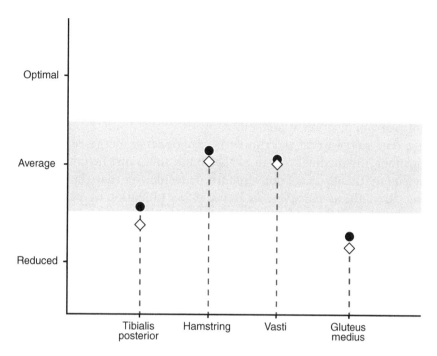

Figure 6.9   Strength measures.
Note: Diamond = right limb; circle = left limb.

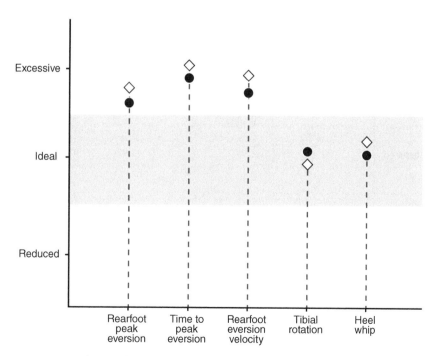

Figure 6.10   Foot biomechanical measures.
Note: Diamond = right limb; circle = left limb.

gluteus medius strength and the slightly high Q-angle measure. Since there is not an excessive amount of knee rotation or hip rotation, the heel whip measure is within normal limits, and sufficient range of motion is measured within the hip rotators (figure 6.12), torsional forces are not playing a significant role in the MTSS pain and symptoms. Figure 6.11 shows that we can visually observe an excessive knee abduction position concomitant with **pelvic drop** and an induced rearfoot eversion position at midstance.

These data suggest that the runner is experiencing increased frontal plane loading along the medial column of the shank that must be counterbalanced with adequate tibialis posterior strength. Considering that the runner lacks adequate strength, we observed the induced foot pronation as the hip and knee collapse drives the foot into this pronated (everted) position. Thus, the MTSS is the direct result of tibialis posterior weakness and increased force output from the muscle because of atypical proximal biomechanics and gluteus medius strength. The MTSS pain is caused by the tibialis posterior muscle pulling away from the medial origin on the tibia and concomitant periositis.

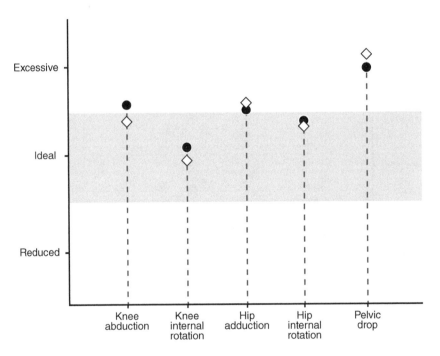

Figure 6.11 Knee and hip biomechanical measures.

Note: Diamond = right limb; circle = left limb.

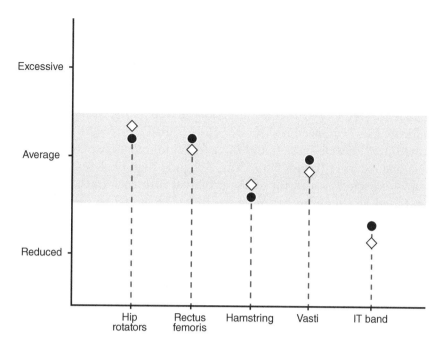

Figure 6.12   Flexibility measures.
Note: Diamond = right limb; circle = left limb.

Assessment Summary

Anatomical

All measures within normal limits

Strength

- Reduced tibialis posterior strength
- Reduced gluteus medius strength

Foot Biomechanics

- Increased peak rearfoot eversion
- Prolonged time to peak rearfoot eversion
- Increased rearfoot eversion velocity

Knee and Hip Biomechanics

- Increased peak knee abduction
- Increased peak hip adduction
- Increased peak pelvic drop

Flexibility

Reduced IT band flexibility

PRIMARY TREATMENT

Primary treatment for this individual includes strengthening of the tibialis posterior and gluteus medius to resolve the excessive and prolonged time to peak rearfoot eversion and high rearfoot eversion velocity. Greater strength will reduce the velocity of rearfoot eversion as well as the knee and hip rotation velocity. However, even if sufficient gluteus medius strength is achieved, a high amount of knee abduction and hip adduction may occur considering the high Q-angle measure (figure 6.8). Thus, a slightly high peak rearfoot eversion position is expected as a result of the proximal influence in this mechanical pattern. Based on this information, a stability shoe would be the ideal shoe to minimize peak excessive rearfoot eversion and control excessive frontal plane forces from a distal aspect. Finally, discontinuing the use of the motion control shoe is necessary considering the typical foot anatomical alignment measures and especially considering the standing rearfoot varus posture.

Focus of Treatment
- Strengthen tibialis posterior
- Strengthen gluteus medius
- Stability shoe
- Discontinue use of motion control shoe

Case Study: Patellofemoral Pain Syndrome

The subject of this case study is a runner presenting with bilateral patellofemoral pain syndrome (PFPS).

 See online videos 6.4*a* and *b* for footage of a runner with patellofemoral pain as described in this case study.

INJURY HISTORY

The runner has retro- and lateropatellar pain near the start of each run and especially when the run ends. Upon clinical inspection, increased crepitus is subjectively determined during the patellar grind test and a patellar apprehension test is negative. Vastus medialis oblique muscle atrophy is not visually observed most likely because the pain and symptoms only manifested themselves over the past 2 months. The runner has not sought treatment elsewhere and has simply tried to manage her pain and symptoms through reduced mileage and icing the affected area after longer runs of 5 to 7 kilometers.

Injury History Summary
Condition
   Bilateral patellofemoral pain syndrome
Duration
   • Less than 2 months
Symptoms
   Retro- and lateropatellar pain
Signs
   • Positive patellar grind test
   • Negative patellar apprehension test
Previous Treatment(s)
   None; self-managed through reduced mileage and ice

ASSESSMENT

All anatomical alignment measures are well within normal limits (figure 6.13). There is a somewhat high forefoot varus orientation along with a somewhat high standing rearfoot valgus posture. Thus, we would expect typical rearfoot eversion from a biomechanical perspective unless significant tibialis posterior muscle weakness is present. Inspection of figure 6.14 shows very good tibialis posterior strength but reduced overall strength in knee and hip musculature.

The average to high ankle invertor (tibialis posterior) strength matches well with the foot biomechanical measures seen in figure 6.15. Overall, typical peak rearfoot eversion and typical rearfoot eversion velocity measures are observed.

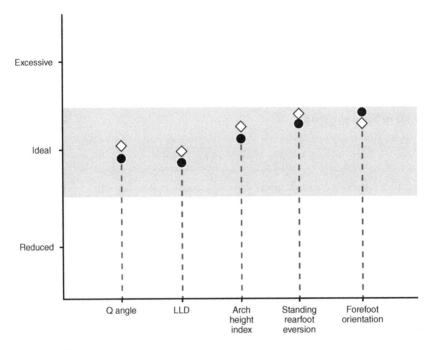

Figure 6.13   Alignment measures.
Note: Diamond = right limb; circle = left limb.

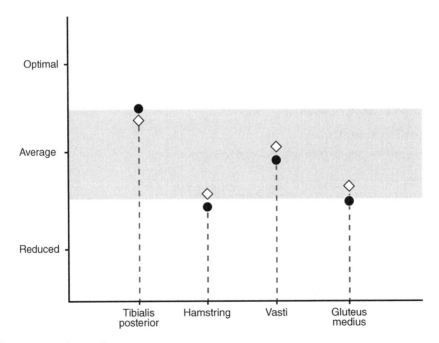

Figure 6.14   Strength measures.
Note: Diamond = right limb; circle = left limb.

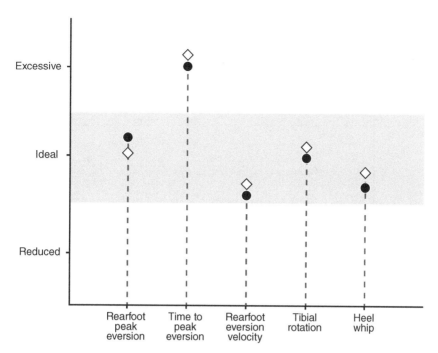

Figure 6.15 Foot biomechanical measures.

Note: Diamond = right limb; circle = left limb.

Ankle invertor muscle strength is what primarily controls the foot, therefore the average to high strength results in the overall typical biomechanical motion. Moreover, the typical tibial internal rotation measures indicate proper coupling of the rearfoot and tibia, suggesting overall distal mechanics are within normal limits. Therefore, the prolonged time to peak rearfoot eversion must be the result of proximal factors.

As seen in figure 6.16, this runner exhibits excessive knee abduction, hip adduction, and contralateral pelvic drop during gait. These increased frontal plane forces can be directly attributed to the lack of gluteus medius muscle strength. The increased frontal plane forces cannot be attributed to any ana-tomical factors considering the Q-angle measure is well within normal limits and all flexibility measures (figure 6.17) are actually reduced, particularly the IT band. In addition, figure 6.16 shows increased knee and hip internal rotation mechanics, which can be attributed to the reduced hamstring, gluteus medius, and hip external rotator strength.

Given the reduced IT band, rectus femoris, and vasti muscles flexibility, the patella may not be articulating properly within the femoral groove as a result of muscle and tissue tightness. Irrespective of this consideration, the PFPS pain and symptoms cannot be primarily attributed to the lack of flexibility. The primary cause of the PFPS symptoms are based on the excessive biomechanical patterns mea-sured, which are primarily attributed to the lack of hip and knee muscle strength. However, the reduced flexibility must be considered within the treatment plan.

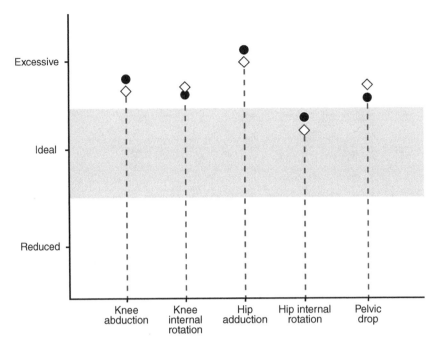

Figure 6.16   Knee and hip biomechanical measures.
Note: Diamond = right limb; circle = left limb.

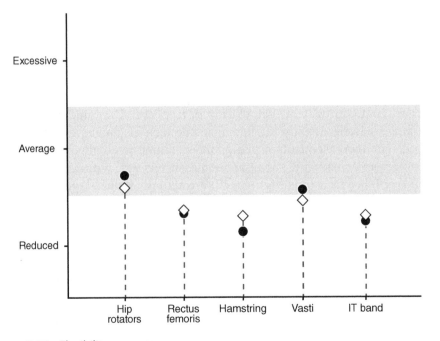

Figure 6.17   Flexibility measures.
Note: Diamond = right limb; circle = left limb.

Assessment Summary

Anatomical
All measures within normal limits

Strength
- Reduced hamstring strength
- Reduced gluteus medius strength

Foot Biomechanics
Prolonged time to peak rearfoot eversion

Knee and Hip Biomechanics
- Increased peak knee abduction
- Increased peak knee internal rotation
- Increased peak hip adduction
- Increased peak pelvic drop

Flexibility
- Reduced rectus femoris flexibility
- Reduced hamstring flexibility
- Reduced vasti flexibility
- Reduced IT band flexibility

PRIMARY TREATMENT

Treatment for this runner includes strengthening of the gluteus medius, hip external rotators, and hamstring musculature to reduce frontal plane and torsional forces at the hip and knee. Since the hamstring is a biarticular muscle, as discussed in chapters 4 and 5, focus should be on knee flexion and hip extension resistance exercises. Moreover, considering the reduced vasti, rectus femoris, and IT band flexibility, efforts towards improving tissue range of motion should also be considered. Considering the typical rearfoot and tibial mechanics, sufficient strength of the tibial posterior muscle, and typical foot alignment measures, this runner should receive a recommendation for a neutral cushioning shoe. An orthotic device is not recommended since peak rearfoot eversion, rearfoot eversion velocity, and peak tibial rotation were all within normal limits from a biomechanical perspective, and all anatomical alignment measures were also within normal limits.

Focus of Treatment
- Strengthen gluteus medius, hip external rotators, and hamstrings
- Increase flexibility of vasti, rectus femoris, and IT band
- Neutral cushioning shoe
- Discontinue use of motion control shoe and orthotics

SUMMARY

Each runner presented with different symptoms and injuries, and each was complex in terms of the interrelationships among the four factors. Yet there were surprising similarities. For example, the runner with tibialis posterior tendinopathy (TPT) the runner with PFPS, and the runner with MTSS exhibited reduced gluteus medius muscle strength. However, the end result was different in that the runner with PFPS and the runner with MTSS exhibited increased peak knee abduction and increased hip adduction, but the TPT runner did not. Moreover, concomitant with the reduced gluteus medius strength, the runner with TPT and the runner with MTSS exhibited increased peak pelvic drop, whereas the PFPS runner did not. Finally, the TPT runner and PFPS runner exhibited reduced hamstring strength, but only the TPT runner also demonstrated increased peak tibial internal rotation as a result. Thus, we can draw two conclusions from these data: First, there is not necessarily a cause-and-effect relationship among the four factors, meaning there are no absolute rules to follow (i.e. reduced gluteus medius strength *always* leads to increased knee abduction), and second, much research is still needed to better develop algorithms for linking these factors together and establishing interrelationships. Regardless, these case studies form a basis from which we can begin to better evaluate and assess gait mechanics and understand injury pathomechanics. The next chapter details some of the research surrounding the question of whether we can change gait mechanics. We'll explore two concepts related to clinical practice: gait retraining and improving muscular strength.

Can We Influence Gait Mechanics?

Abnormal running mechanics are often cited as the cause of running-related injuries and many attempts have been made to alter a patient's mechanical pattern to reduce or alter the loads experienced by the tissues and joint of interest. For example, as discussed in chapter 3, foot orthotic devices are commonly used to attempt to modify abnormal running mechanics. If improper mechanics are the cause of an injury, when the patient returns to running, the problem will likely reoccur. However, few sports medicine professionals suggest altering the running pattern to reduce the risk of injury. In part, this is because locomotion is thought to be automatic and thus difficult to change.

From a historical perspective, therapists, coaches, and clinicians have worked to alter movement patterns to increase performance and decrease injury. Indeed, if a runner is able to modify their gait patterns and correct the abnormal mechanics, the risk for further injury is likely to be reduced.

FEEDBACK

There have been numerous reports in the literature documenting the success of using some type of feedback training to alter gait. The majority of these reports focus on patients with neurologic involvement, such as adults who have sustained a stroke or children with cerebral palsy. The earliest forms of feedback were limb load monitors placed within the shoe of a patient (Wannstedt and Herman 1978; Seeger et al. 1981; Seeger and Caudrey 1983). The aim of this type of feedback was to produce an equal load distribution between lower extremities during gait. EMG is another form of feedback that reports improvements in gait symmetry in terms of spatio-temporal parameters and joint motion patterns. (Burnside et al. 1982; Colborne et al. 1993; Colborne et al. 1994; Intiso et al. 1994). Finally, feedback on joint angles has been provided through the use of electrogoniometers for patients with **genu recurvatum** (Hogue and McCandless 1983; Olney et al. 1989; Morris et al. 1992). An overwhelming majority of these studies have reported successful results. However, these techniques have not been widely reported on in the biomechanics literature.

Visual Feedback

In a case study, McClay et al. (1999) reported that visual feedback, provided by a mirror, produced quantitative changes in a runner with a history of plantar fasciitis. The patient presented with a common misalignment syndrome, involving excessive hip adduction and internal rotation and knee abduction. She also presented with hip abduction and external rotator weakness and excessive hip internal rotation range. After 8 weeks of feedback training, the patient was able to decrease her hip adduction and internal rotation as well as her knee abduction and rotation. These alterations led to a resolution of her symptoms. In addition, she maintained most of the changes 6 months later after termination of the feedback training. With the advent of real-time motion analysis, the mirror can now be replaced with a computer monitor. Markers are placed on segments of the lower extremity and any of the three dimension components of motion at any joint can be visualized on the screen. Through the use of targets, patients can use their real-time joint angles to improve their mechanics. There has been some research aimed at better understanding the clinical efficacy of real-time feedback and modifying gait mechanics.

Real-Time Feedback

Several studies have been published regarding the use of real-time feedback and alterations in biomechanical running patterns. Crowell and Davis (2011) recruited 10 runners who exhibited peak positive tibial acceleration greater than 8 g, as measured using an accelerometer. Baseline biomechanical data were collected, and the runners began the retraining sessions, which included eight sessions over a 2-week period. The accelerometer was taped to the distal aspect of the runner's tibia, and the signal from the accelerometer was displayed on a monitor in front of the treadmill. Subjects were instructed to run softer by making their footfalls quieter and keep the acceleration peaks below a 4 g mark shown on the screen. After the retraining, the peak acceleration was reduced by 50% and the vertical force loading rates and the vertical force impact peak were approximately 30% and 20% lower, respectively. These authors reported that at a 1-month follow-up these altered loading patterns were still apparent and concluded that this type of feedback training might reduce the runner's potential for developing stress fractures. However, no further follow-up was provided.

Barrios et al. (2010) investigated whether the knee adduction moment, the torque produced to resist knee abduction movement pattern during gait, can be reduced. This type of study may be important since varus alignment and high knee adduction loading have been linked to the development of osteoarthritis (Brouwer et al. 2007). Eight healthy, varus-aligned individuals underwent a gait retraining protocol over a 1-month period. As a subject walked on an instrumented treadmill, their frontal plane knee angle was displayed in real time for feedback. After the retraining sessions, an 8° increase in hip internal rotation, a 3° increase in hip adduction, a 2° reduction in knee adduction angles, and an 18% decrease in the knee adduction moment were reported. Based on these alterations, the authors concluded that a gait retraining may be a powerful approach to reduce medial knee joint loading during gait.

Finally, Noehren et al. (2011) investigated whether real-time feedback improves hip mechanics and reduces pain in subjects with PFPS. Real-time kinematic feedback of peak hip adduction angle was provided for 10 runners over eight training sessions. After the protocol, hip internal rotation decreased by 21%, hip adduction decreased by 18%, and ground reaction loading rates decreased by 20%. There was also a significant reduction in PFPS pain and improvements in function after the protocol.

It is well accepted that abnormal mechanics play a role in running injuries. Unfortunately, there are only a handful of research studies investigating whether real-time feedback can alter running and walking patterns and whether these alterations lead to reduced pain and improved function. Overall, the results of these studies are positive and suggest that this approach is beneficial for rehabilitation and possibly for prevention of injury reoccurrence.

However, there are no long-term follow-up studies to insure that these alterations can be maintained over a long period of time and, more important, that these alterations do not lead to other musculoskeletal injuries. Changing one factor, albeit an important factor such as movement biomechanics, should only be done when the factors of strength, flexibility, and anatomical alignment have been considered and evaluated. On one hand, it is easy to argue that if atypical mechanics are not altered, the injury is likely to reoccur. However, one could also argue that redistribution of loading simply leads to other injuries. Various types of feedback training have been used widely and successfully for neurologic patients with gait problems. However, altering the gait patterns of injured runners has not received much attention.

STRENGTH TRAINING

In contrast to using motion capture, ground reaction force, or accelerometer data to change a runner's movement pattern, there has been some research concerning alterations of movement patterns through strength training. Snyder et al. (2009) reported that after a 6-week hip strengthening protocol, healthy female runners exhibited a 13% gain in abductor strength, but the hip adduction angle during running increased by 1.4°, contrary to their hypotheses and the concepts discussed in chapter 5. Earl and Hoch (2011) recruited 19 women runners currently experiencing PFPS, and they participated in an 8-week program to strengthen the hip and core musculature. After the protocol, significant improvements in pain, function, and muscle strength were reported. There were significant improvements in the knee adduction moment, but no changes in peak knee or hip joint angles were reported, suggesting that knee joint loading was reduced with increased muscle strength.

As discussed in chapter 4, we conducted a study involving 15 individuals with PFPS who participated in a 3-week hip strengthening protocol. Compared to baseline values, all 15 PFPS subjects exhibited increases in muscle strength, 13 of the 15 PFPS patients exhibited reductions in stride-to-stride knee joint variability, and 13 of the 15 patients reported at least a 33% decrease in pain as measured by a Visual Analog Scale (VAS: a 10 cm scale) over the course of the study. In fact, 4 of the PFPS patients reported being pain-free at the end of the 3 weeks. Thus, we concluded that a 3-week hip abductor muscle strengthening protocol is effective in increasing muscle strength, decreasing stride-to-stride knee joint variability, and decreasing the level of pain experienced by individuals with PFPS. The results of this study also suggest that stride-to-stride knee joint variability may be a better indicator of injury rehabilitation progression compared to peak angles.

REVISITING THE CASE STUDIES

The majority of the treatment recommendations provided in chapter 6 were to increase muscle strength and concomitantly alter running gait mechanics via reducing peak joint angles. However, alterations in gait mechanics can occur through the use of real-time feedback.

For example, the runner with TPT and the runner with MTSS could have benefited from gait retraining that focused on reducing the amount of hip and tibial rotation. One could accomplish this by running in a more toed-in position, but this would counteract the concept of gait retraining and could result in other torsional stresses as the toed-in position is atypical. Thus, using a mirror and having the runner focus on gluteal contractions through verbal instruction is the method of choice. Using phrases such as "squeeze your gluteals together" and having runners focus on maintaining the tibial tuberosity in an anterior direction (while maintaining their typical foot progression angle, or their **toe-out angle**) is recommended. This complex task requires training and practice.

Another example involves the runner with PFPS. The frontal plane mechanics exhibited by this runner could be resolved by asking her to maintain a more vertical frontal plane knee and hip position possibly through a slight increase in step width and through gluteal muscle activation. Having the runner focus on hamstring activation at heel strike and throughout the gait cycle would serve to improve knee joint stability as well.

In light of these gait-retraining recommendations, and in our clinical opinion, gait retraining and muscle strengthening can be more powerful and efficacious when performed together. However, there is no research to support or refute one method over the other. Regardless, a combined approach that allows the patient to focus on daily rehabilitation is the most effective. For example, a patient with a running-related injury would never run every day to retrain their gait mechanics, and the gait-retraining research involves 2 or 3 days per week of gait retraining over a period of 6 to 8 weeks. Thus, the other 4 or 5 days per week could be focused on muscle strengthening for optimal results.

SUMMARY

There is evidence to suggest that gait retraining using real-time feedback can alter gait patterns and reduce pain. However, there is also evidence that muscle strengthening can accomplish the same goal. While one method cannot be stated as being superior to the other, they are effective and available to clinicians for rehabilitation of their patients. The clinician must make an evidence-based decision about which treatment modality (or whether both options) optimizes treatment outcomes and reduces the potential for reinjury.

Overview of Clinical and Biomechanical Assessment

Now that we have discussed many interrelationships among various clinical and biomechanical factors, we hope you are gaining an appreciation for the complexity of comprehensive analysis of the entire lower extremity. In an attempt to simplify the process of establishing these interrelationships, this chapter provides several tables that show how these factors relate to one another. We call the collection of tables our road map because we constantly refer to them to help guide us through interpreting and understanding our patients and their associated pathomechanics.

We have chosen to use observable or measurable biomechanical factors as the frame of reference to help guide and assist in musculoskeletal injury assessment. Moreover, the anatomical alignment, strength, and flexibility factors discussed directly relate to those in earlier chapters. If, for example, we do not list any flexibility factors, it is because there is no literature to validate its relationship to the biomechanical variables discussed. For other variables, such as peak knee flexion, there are no anatomical alignment factors related which we can discuss. This is either because there is little or no research or because we consider it to be a nonfactor in determining the overall movement pattern. First, we start with the foot and move up the kinematic chain.

FOOT, ANKLE, AND TIBIA

For the foot, ankle, and tibia, we have listed those structural, strength, and flexibility factors we discussed in the previous chapters. These are grouped into tables by biomechanical pattern. Not all factors listed in the right-hand column will be present for any given person with that atypical movement pattern. Excessive and reduced peak rearfoot eversion are listed as both being associated with injury. Excessive peak eversion velocity and excessive time to peak rearfoot eversion are also listed, but we do not discuss reduced eversion velocity or reduced (early) time to peak eversion as there is nothing in the scientific literature. We do not consider a low eversion velocity movement to be potentially injurious either. Finally, we've listed those factors associated with excessive and reduced peak tibial internal rotation, and it should become clear how proximal biomechanical factors are associated with these motions.

Excessive Peak Rearfoot Eversion

Anatomical alignment	Increased rearfoot valgus standing angle Forefoot varus orientation Low arch height index or change in arch height measure
Strength	Reduced tibialis posterior strength
Flexibility	Increased first ray dorsiflexion range of motion
Biomechanics	1. Associated with increased hip adduction and knee abduction causing an induced increase in peak rearfoot eversion 2. Coupled motion with tibial internal rotation, resulting in increased tibial and knee internal rotation

Reduced Peak Rearfoot Eversion

Anatomical alignment	Rearfoot varus standing angle Forefoot valgus orientation High arch height index or change in arch height measure
Strength	—
Flexibility	Reduced gastrocnemius and soleus range of motion Reduced first ray range of motion
Biomechanics	1. Associated with reduced hip adduction and knee abduction 2. Coupled motion with tibial internal rotation, resulting in reduced tibial and knee internal rotation

Excessive Rearfoot Eversion Velocity

Anatomical alignment	—
Strength	Reduced tibialis posterior strength
Flexibility	—
Biomechanics	Associated with increased hip adduction and knee abduction, causing induced peak rearfoot eversion

Prolonged Time to Peak Rearfoot Eversion

Anatomical alignment	Increased rearfoot valgus standing angle Forefoot varus orientation Low arch height index or change in arch height measure
Strength	Reduced tibialis posterior strength
Flexibility	—
Biomechanics	1. Associated with increased hip adduction and knee abduction, causing induced peak rearfoot eversion 2. Coupled motion with tibial internal rotation, resulting in increased tibial and knee internal rotation

Excessive Peak Tibial Internal Rotation

Anatomical alignment	—
Strength	Reduced tibialis posterior, hamstring, hip external rotator strength
Flexibility	—
Biomechanics	Associated with increased peak rearfoot eversion, eversion velocity, knee internal rotation

Reduced Peak Tibial Internal Rotation

Anatomical alignment	Rearfoot varus standing angle Forefoot valgus orientation High arch height index or change in arch height measure
Strength	—
Flexibility	Reduced lateral soft tissue range of motion, such as in the IT band, biceps femoris, gastrocnemius, or soleus
Biomechanics	Coupled motion with foot pronation, resulting in reduced peak rearfoot eversion

KNEE

When discussing atypical knee gait mechanics we begin to make links to both distal and proximal biomechanical factors. In these tables we discuss excessive peak knee abduction (genu valgum) and reduced knee abduction (genu varum) with links to rearfoot, hip, and pelvis. Thus, a local biomechanical pattern that is atypical can be attributed to a distal or a proximal factor. We also discuss excessive and reduced peak knee internal rotation but only excessive peak knee flexion.

Excessive Peak Knee Abduction

Anatomical alignment	Increased Q-angle
Strength	Reduced hip abductor, external rotator (gluteus medius), or hamstring strength
Flexibility	—
Biomechanics	1. Associated with excessive hip adduction or internal rotation, knee internal rotation, and pelvic drop 2. Associated with excessive peak rearfoot eversion or prolonged peak rearfoot eversion

Reduced Peak Knee Abduction

Anatomical alignment	Reduced Q-angle
Strength	—
Flexibility	—
Biomechanics	1. Associated with reduced hip adduction or internal rotation, knee internal rotation, and pelvic drop 2. Associated with reduced peak rearfoot eversion

Excessive Peak Knee Internal Rotation

Anatomical alignment	—
Strength	Reduced hamstring or gluteus medius strength
Flexibility	—
Biomechanics	1. Associated excessive peak rearfoot eversion and hip or tibial internal rotation 2. Associated with increased heel whip or prolonged pronation

Reduced Peak Knee Internal Rotation

Anatomical alignment	Supinated (cavus) foot static posture
Strength	—
Flexibility	Reduced lateral soft tissue range of motion, such as IT band, biceps femoris, gastrocnemius, or soleus
Biomechanics	1. Associated reduced peak rearfoot eversion and hip or tibial internal rotation 2. Associated with decreased peak rearfoot eversion

Excessive Peak Knee Flexion

Anatomical alignment	—
Strength	Reduced hamstring or vasti muscle strength
Flexibility	—
Biomechanics	Increased tibial and knee internal rotation, increased peak rearfoot eversion

HIP

Our final tables discuss excessive and reduced peak hip adduction and internal rotation and excessive pelvic drop. At this point many interrelationships should be clear, but not all factors are necessarily related to one another. For example, excessive rearfoot eversion may be a consequence of excessive knee abduction, and excessive hip adduction may not be present. Alternatively, an excessive Q-angle may be present and the sole contributor to excessive knee abduction.

Excessive Peak Hip Adduction

Anatomical alignment	Increased Q-angle
Strength	Weakness of gluteus medius muscle
Flexibility	—
Biomechanics	1. Associated with excessive peak knee abduction and contralateral pelvic drop 2. Can be associated with excessive peak hip internal rotation and excessive or prolonged rearfoot eversion

Reduced Peak Hip Adduction

Anatomical alignment	Decreased Q-angle
Strength	—
Flexibility	Reduced IT band flexibility
Biomechanics	1. Associated with reduced peak knee abduction and contralateral pelvic drop 2. Can be associated with reduced peak hip internal rotation and reduced rearfoot eversion

Excessive Peak Hip Internal Rotation

Anatomical alignment	—
Strength	Weakness of hip abductor and external rotator muscle
Flexibility	Increased hip internal rotator range of motion
Biomechanics	1. Associated with increased heel whip and foot progression angle 2. Associated with excessive peak hip adduction and tibial or knee internal rotation

Reduced Peak Hip Internal Rotation

Anatomical alignment	—
Strength	—
Flexibility	Reduced hip internal rotator range of motion
Biomechanics	1. Associated with decreased heel whip and foot progression angle 2. Associated with decreased peak hip adduction and tibial or knee internal rotation

Excessive Peak Pelvic Drop

Anatomical alignment	—
Strength	Reduced contralateral hip abductor stabilizer and overall core strength
Flexibility	—
Biomechanics	Associated with excessive hip adduction or internal rotation and knee abduction

SUMMARY

There are still many unanswered questions about running biomechanics and kinetic-chain interrelationships that have not been answered in the scientific literature. One excellent example is the tibial and femoral torsion caused by some runners' anatomical structure and this pattern's relationship to hip and knee rotation. At the Running Injury Clinic we have been investigating these factors but have yet to draw firm conclusions. Our central hypothesis is that excessive tibial torsion, or a more externally rotated tibia, is related to decreased knee internal rotation and a more toed-out foot progression angle when running, which can lead to increased torsional stress. In accordance, we hypothesize that excessive femoral torsion, or a more internally rotated femur often called anteversion, is related to decreased hip internal rotation. While these seem like reasonable hypotheses, they have not been tested empirically and have thus not been included in these tables or within this textbook. As research advances and these interrelationships become clearer, they will be added and discussed.

Chapter 9 discusses technical aspects of video gait analysis from a 2D perspective. While 3D motion capture is considered the gold standard (and therefore we presented 3D data in case studies and research presented in this book), clinicians generally do not have access to complex 3D motion capture systems, so single camera systems are often used in the clinical setting. We present several technical aspects to help optimize the use of a single camera for the purpose of clinical gait analysis.

Technical Aspects of Video Gait Analysis

Screening for excessive atypical movement patterns during walking or running can help facilitate effective clinical interventions and aid in injury prevention. Clinicians do not generally have access to complex 3D motion capture systems. So single camera, 2D camera systems are often used in the clinical setting for their practicality because they require fewer markers, are less expensive, and use less space than multicamera, 3D motion analysis systems. However, 3D camera systems, the gold standard for motion analysis, allow for the assessment of multiplanar motion, and the higher-frequency cameras offer greater precision for tracking motion. Thus, understanding the relationship between 2D and 3D motion systems allows research findings to be more applicable to the clinical setting and provide a better understanding of the potential error associated with a 2D system.

Studies have investigated the relationship between 2D and 3D motion capture for gait biomechanics. The first study published by Areblad et al. (1990) concluded that "[it is advisable to] use a three-dimensional model when studying motion between foot and lower leg during running" (p. 933). A follow-up study by McClay and Manal (1998) investigated 2D error produced by varying amounts of foot and camera positions and concluded that "caution should be exercised when assessing two-dimensional rearfoot motion" (p. 26). A more recent paper by McLean et al. (2003) reported that errors in the magnitude of 200% were present when comparing 2D angles to 3D angles during side step, side jump, and shuttle run but that the waveform pattern between 2D and 3D are similar. Our research (Cormack et al. 2011) verifies these findings and demonstrates a consistent overestimation of hip and knee measurements using a 2D approach.

Based on these studies, it can be concluded that a 3D approach to gait analysis is superior and should be considered the gold standard. However, 3D systems are generally cost prohibitive, involve technical skills and training to operate, and take time to process the data. Thus, we discuss how to optimize a 2D approach for recording gait biomechanics. Several factors must be considered when determining the ideal equipment based on a 2D data collection including, but not limited to, cost, portability, software, and sampling rate.

SAMPLING FREQUENCY

With respect to **sampling frequency** (or sometimes referred to as sampling rate), a camera system with a high **collection frequency** is desirable based on the need to capture the higher-frequency movement associated with jerky pathological gait. Sampling frequency is measured in Hertz and refers to the number of frames of data collected every second. For example, 30 Hz means 30 frames of data are collected every second.

The minimum sampling rate required is determined using the **sampling theorem**, which states that any signal should be sampled at least twice the rate of the highest frequency inherent in the signal itself (Winter 1990). If movement data are collected at too low a frequency, aliasing errors are present, resulting in false frequencies that were not present in the original signal. Thus, errors in the detection of specific gait events as well as kinematic measurements occur and lead to an inability to accurately measure the joint angle.

During a clinical gait assessment, there is considerable evidence that human movement contains frequencies up to 6 Hertz (Hz: 1 cycle per second) and that insignificant frequency components are present above that threshold (Winter 1982; Polk 2005). For example, during walking gait, stride frequency is less than 1 Hz, and during running it is approximately 4 Hz. Thus, the use of expensive, higher-speed cameras may not be warranted depending on what gait parameters were selected for the research or clinical question. However, the determination of a specific gait event, such as heel strike and heel lift, is critical for measuring specific gait patterns and these events occur at a very high frequency. Thus, use of a high-speed camera is warranted.

We conducted a study to determine the differences in measurements of common gait events and rearfoot measures using a standard 30 Hz digital camera compared to a 100 Hz high-speed camera (Ferber et al. 2009). We simultaneously collected 2D data using the two different cameras from 10 recreational runners who demonstrated a heel strike pattern. We thought this was an important study because no previous research study had specifically quantified the measurement differences for common rearfoot clinical gait variables between different camera systems. Often, a clinician or researcher is faced with an economic or a scientific dilemma with respect to purchasing an expensive kinematic data collection system to provide accurate data to determine the optimal treatment for a patient or for accuracy of results. This study would serve to establish the technical requirements for conducting an in-clinic 2D gait analysis.

The results of the study show that the average measurement differences were between 6.6% to 14.3% of the stance phase of running gait for temporal variables (determining heel strike and heel lift) and errors of 1.02° for rearfoot eversion were measured for a 30 Hz camera compared to a 100 Hz camera (figure 9.1).

Figure 9.1 is a representation of a typical footfall used for analysis in both the time domain and magnitude of rearfoot eversion comparing the 30 Hz camera and the 100 Hz camera. Maximum rearfoot eversion for the 30 Hz camera occurred at 48% of stance (or 120 ms after heel strike) while maximum rearfoot eversion for the 100 Hz camera occurred at 45% of stance (or 112 ms after heel strike) resulting in an 8 ms difference. In other words, the 30 Hz camera did not accurately reflect when the foot actually struck the ground. Figure 9.1 also demonstrates the difference in the maximum rearfoot eversion value equating to a 1.02° difference between cameras, showing that the 30 Hz camera overestimated the actual amount of rearfoot eversion. Finally, in figure 9.1 it can be observed that there is no data for the 30 Hz camera for the first 5% of stance, which is an example of the reported 11.9% average difference in determining

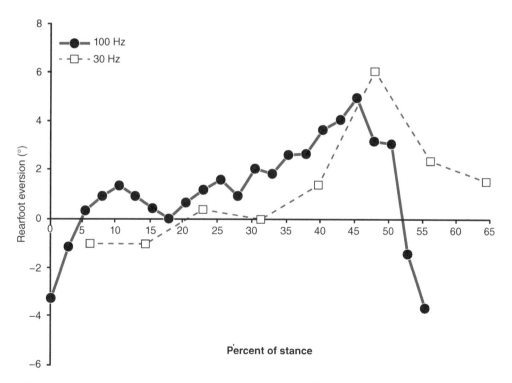

Figure 9.1 Representative graph of a typical footfall used for analysis from the 30 Hz camera and the 100 Hz camera for the percentage of the gait cycle from heel strike to heel lift.

"Measurement error of rearfoot kinematics during running between a 100Hz and 30Hz camera," R. Ferber, K. Sheerin and K. Kendall, *International SportMed Journal*, 10(3):152-162. Copyright 2009. Reproduced by permission of International SportMed Journal.

heel strike error wherein the 30 Hz camera missed the actual frame of heel strike compared to the 100 Hz camera.

When making a decision to purchase a camera for the purpose of biomechanical gait analysis, a 100 Hz camera should be considered the minimum collection frequency to produce as accurate results as possible using a 2D approach.

F-STOP AND SHUTTER SPEED

When recording a biomechanical gait pattern, the f-stop, or the aperture opening, is an important consideration. The aperture is a hole or an opening in the lens of the camera through which light travels, and it plays an important role in terms of the sharpness of the image being recorded. The easiest way to picture the aperture is that it is similar to the iris and pupil in your eye. The iris, or aperture, opens and closes to allow more or less light inside the lens (the pupil). The camera lens aperture is specified as an f-number, or f-stop, which is the ratio of focal length to aperture diameter. In other words, a high f-stop number means that the aperture is smaller, allowing less light to enter. A small f-stop number means that the aperture is wider, allowing more light inside the camera. However, keep in mind that for each setting that the aperture is reduced, the volume of light passing through the lens is cut in half. Finally, consider that the depth of field is influenced by the f-stop value: A low f-number tends to have subjects at one distance in focus, while objects nearer and farther away are out of focus.

Shutter speed is another important consideration. It is important to remember that shutter speed and sampling frequency are two different considerations. Sampling frequency (rate) refers to the number of frames of data collected every second. Shutter speed refers to the amount of time that the volume of light coming through the lens (determined by the aperture or f-stop value) is allowed to stay on the film or digital media in the camera. Generally shutter speed is denoted as the inverse of 1 second: 1/500 indicates that the shutter stays open for 1/500 of a second, or 0.002 second. The longer the shutter speed, the more time light has to enter the camera and be recorded. Conversely, the shorter the shutter speed, the less time light has to enter. Thus, a high shutter speed requires a larger aperture, or f-stop setting, to ensure sufficient light exposure, whereas a low shutter speed requires a smaller aperture to avoid excessive exposure.

Generally, running gait involves fast motions of the individual joints and segments and thus requires a fast collection frequency (minimum 100 Hz), a fast shutter speed, and a larger aperture. These settings together also require sufficient external light to ensure a sharp image to help improve the accuracy of the data.

SOFTWARE OPTIONS

Many different software options for 2D video analysis are available, including Dartfish (www.dartfish.com), Silicon Coach (www.siliconcoach.com), Sports Motion (www.sportsmotion.com), and Mar-Systems (www.mar-systems.co.uk). Unfortunately, no research studies have been conducted regarding measurement error across multiple software platforms. The aforementioned study by McLean et al. (2003) that compared 2D to 3D measures involved a free 2D software program called DgeeMe 1.0 (www.freedownloadscenter.com/Multimedia_and_Graphics/Video_and_Animation_Tools/DgeeMe.html) and the manual selection of the points of interest on a frame-by-frame basis. To our knowledge, the only 2D software that is commercially available and has an auto-labeling function is Vicon Motus (www.motus10.com). While auto-labeling has the advantage of being less time consuming, the error as compared to manual digitization is unknown.

SUMMARY

Based on the review of literature that has investigated 2D and 3D gait biomechanics and the errors associated with 2D analysis, clinicians should be aware that no matter what 2D software package they purchase, errors in excess of 30% may be present when attempting to calculate joint angles using a 2D approach. While 3D motion capture systems are considered the gold standard, 2D errors can be minimized by using a 100 Hz camera, having appropriate lighting, and adjusting the f-stop and shutter speed accordingly. Moreover, any atypical biomechanics measured, whether through a 2D or 3D approach, should be combined and considered with respect to muscle strength, anatomical alignment, and tissue flexibility for a comprehensive evaluation of gait pathomechanics.

Afterword

While the title of the book is *Running Mechanics and Gait Analysis*, we hope that our goal of providing a thorough understanding of the complexities of running biomechanics and the interrelationships of muscular strength, flexibility, and anatomical alignment has been met. Advanced clinical gait assessment is a complex process and too often a subjective process. Our hope is that the information in this book regarding the research behind the interrelationships among variables and the evidence-based values related to typical and atypical values is incorporated into clinical practices and daily running regimens. All of the theories put forth are grounded in the most current biomechanical and clinical research to provide innovative tools to help improve clinical practices and the ability to rehabilitate and prevent injuries. Happy running!

Appendix
Terminology for Gait Biomechanics

Foot Complex

peak rearfoot eversion: How much the foot collapses inward when running and a component of overall foot pronation. Pronation is synonymous to the foot unlocking and is necessary to accommodate uneven surfaces, dissipate impact forces, and allow the big toe to reach the ground. Excessive rearfoot eversion can cause the lower leg to rotate too far inward, which may increase twisting forces at the ankle and knee. Reduced foot pronation means the foot does not unlock and thereby does not reduce the shock wave of force traveling from the foot upward, resulting in increased stress to the body. Excessive rearfoot eversion is also linked to excessive knee abduction and hip adduction.

rearfoot eversion velocity: How quickly the rearfoot everts. If eversion and overall foot pronation occur too quickly, the lower leg rotates inward too quickly, and the result is increased twisting forces at the ankle and knee. Reduced eversion velocity is not considered to be a clinically relevant measure.

time to peak rearfoot eversion: The amount of time it takes for the rearfoot to reach maximum eversion, which should occur around 50% of stance. The foot needs to completely pronate, the big toe needs to get on the ground, and then the foot needs to begin to supinate (lock up) to form a rigid lever. The supinated foot position produces a rigid lever in preparation for toe-off and maintains overall joint alignment. If the foot stays pronated for too long, twisting forces at the ankle and knee joint can occur. If the foot pronates too quickly, an increase in the shock wave of force traveling from the foot upward occurs, resulting in increased stress to the body.

peak tibial internal rotation: How much the lower leg (shank, or tibia and fibula) rotates inward. This motion is mechanically coupled with rearfoot eversion as well as hip and knee internal rotation. Too much or too little internal rotation creates increased twisting forces to the ankle and knee.

tibial internal rotation velocity: How quickly the lower leg rotates inward. The velocity of inward rotation is mechanically coupled with rearfoot eversion as well as hip and knee internal rotation velocity. Rotation that occurs too quickly or not quickly enough creates increased twisting forces to the ankle and knee.

Knee Complex

peak knee abduction: The amount the knee collapses inward (genu valgum). This is a typical motion when running and is mechanically coupled with rearfoot eversion and hip adduction. It is also coupled with hip and knee internal rotation. Too much knee abduction results in increased stress to the knee joint, the patella (knee cap), and the lower leg.

knee abduction velocity: How quickly the knee collapses inward. If the knee collapses inward too quickly, it can result in increased stress to the knee joint, the patella (knee cap), and the lower leg. Reduced knee-abduction velocity is not considered to be a clinically relevant measure.

peak knee internal rotation: The amount the knee rotates inward. This is a typical motion when running and is mechanically coupled with tibial and hip internal rotation. It is also coupled with hip and knee abduction. Too much internal rotation results in increased stress to the knee joint, the patella (knee cap), and the lower leg.

peak knee flexion: The amount the knee flexes during running. A certain amount of flexion is needed to help dissipate the shock wave traveling up the leg from the foot. Significant side-to-side difference in the amount of knee flexion is a good indicator of an antalgic (limping) gait pattern.

Hip Complex

peak hip adduction: How much the hip collapses inward. This motion is coupled with hip and knee internal rotation as well as knee abduction (collapse inward). A greater than normal amount of inward collapse can contribute to increased forces within the pelvis, hip, and knee joints. Increased hip collapse can also force the knee inward and create an induced (excessive) rearfoot eversion position or cause it to stay in an everted position for too long.

peak hip internal rotation: How much the hip rotates inward. This motion is coupled with knee and tibial internal rotation as well as hip adduction. Increased inward rotation can contribute to increased twisting forces in the pelvis, hip, and knee joints.

peak pelvic drop: How much the hip drops on the opposite side of the single-support leg. With each step during gait, there is time spent standing on one leg, which is called single support. During single support, the pelvis, opposite to the stance limb, drops slightly. Excessive pelvic drop is associated with excessive hip adduction and knee abduction on the opposite (contralateral) side of the body and can create increased shearing forces in the pelvis, hip, and low back.

Functional Outcomes

stride width: The side-to-side distance between left and right footsteps. A narrow stride width is indicative of a crossover foot-strike pattern requiring compensatory hip-stabilizer muscle strength to counterbalance the increased forces. Narrow stride width is also associated with increased rearfoot eversion and tibial internal rotation velocity as well as reduced time to peak rearfoot eversion. Increased stride width is not considered to be a clinically relevant measure.

stride rate: The number of strides (footstrike to footstrike) taken with each foot every minute. This number depends on the speed of running and leg length. There is no ideal stride rate, but significant side-to-side differences are a good indicator of an antalgic gait pattern.

foot progression angle: The amount the foot angles out or in while it is on the ground (i.e., duck-footed or pigeon-toed.) Typically, the foot is turned outward while standing due to anatomical alignment. When running, however, the foot needs to be pointed more straightforward or slightly inward to reduce loading at the knee joint. A reduced or increased foot progression angle is needed to compensate for atypical hip, knee, and tibial rotation and rotation velocity. Significant side-to-side differences are a good indicator of an antalgic gait pattern.

Glossary

collection frequency—Synonymous with sampling rate, the number of frames of data collected every second. For example, 30 Hz means 30 frames of data are collected every second.

coupling variability—The relative angles (motion) between two adjacent joints or segments when discussing local variability; a combination of between-limb or within-limb kinematic patterns for the purpose of a movement goal when discussing global variability.

curved last—The amount of curvature for the shoe as measured by the long axis of the forefoot compared to the long axis of the rearfoot. A semicurved last refers to greater than 5° angulation inward between the forefoot and rearfoot.

foot flare—The amount of curvature for the foot as measured by the long axis of the forefoot compared to the long axis of the rearfoot. Most people exhibit a foot flare angle between 3° and 5°, which corresponds to a semicurved shoe last.

forefoot valgus—A structural component of the foot in which the forefoot is everted with respect to a neutral rearfoot.

forefoot varus—A structural component of the foot in which the forefoot is inverted with respect to a neutral rearfoot.

frontal plane motion—Movement that occurs away or toward the midline of the body. For example, when observing a runner from behind, rearfoot eversion and knee abduction (genu valgum) occur along the frontal plane.

f-stop—A high f-stop number means that the aperture is narrow, allowing less light. A small f-stop number means that the aperture is wider, allowing more light inside the camera. The aperture opening is a hole or an opening in the lens of the camera through which light travels. It plays an important role in terms of the sharpness of the image being recorded.

genu valgum (knee abduction)—The amount the knee collapses inward. This is a typical motion when running and is mechanically coupled with foot pronation and hip adduction. It is also coupled with hip and knee internal rotation. Too much inward collapse results in increased stress to the knee joint, the patella, and lower leg.

genu recurvatum—Hyperextension, or backward angulation of the knee.

heel whip—During gait, the hip and knee internally rotate, creating torsional forces. Once the foot comes off of the ground, the leg rotates outward much like a spring that is allowed to unwind. A typical amount of heel whip, or unwinding, occurs for every runner. However, with insufficient flexibility or strength, an increased whip is observed, indicating increased twisting forces within the ankle, knee, and hip and that the spring was wound too tight during each step.

hip adduction—The amount of femoral adduction which occurs relative to a neutral pelvis. This motion is coupled with hip and knee internal rotation as well as knee abduction during gait. A greater than normal amount of inward hip adduction can contribute to increased forces within the pelvis, hip, and knee joints. Increased hip adduction can also force the knee inward and induce an excessive foot pronation position or cause increased time to peak pronation.

hip extension—The amount of femoral extension at push-off. A certain amount of extension is needed to help dissipate the shock wave traveling up the leg from the foot and to maintain forward velocity, thereby reducing the impact forces during the next step or footstrike. Significant side-to-side difference in the amount of hip extension is an indicator of an antalgic (limping) gait pattern.

hip rotation—The amount of rotation about the long axis of the femur. This motion is coupled with knee and tibial internal rotation as well as hip adduction. Increased inward rotation can contribute to increased torsional forces within the pelvis, hip, and knee joints.

joint coupling—A combination of between-limb or within-limb biomechanical movement patterns for the purpose of an overall movement goal. Joint coupling can be considered local, defined as the coupling or relative movement between joints (ankle and knee) or segments (shank and thigh), or global, defined as whole body coordination of movement patterns.

knee abduction (genu valgum)—The amount the knee collapses inward. This is a typical motion when running and is mechanically coupled with foot pronation and hip adduction. It is also coupled with hip and knee internal rotation. Too much inward collapse results in increased stress to the knee joint, the patella, and lower leg.

knee flexion—The amount the femur moves toward the lower leg, or shank, in stance phase during running. A certain amount of flexion at foot strike is needed to help dissipate the shock wave traveling up the leg from the foot. Significant side-to-side difference in the amount of knee flexion is an indicator of an antalgic gait pattern.

knee rotation—The amount the tibia rotates inward on the femur. This is a typical motion when running and is mechanically coupled with ankle and hip internal rotation as well as hip adduction and knee abduction. Too much internal rotation results in increased stress to the knee joint, the patella, and lower leg.

motion control shoe—A running shoe with a significant amount of foot pronation control and often with some type of nondeformable material, such as a plastic plug, placed on the posteromedial aspect of the shoe. This type of shoe has little cushioning material and is designed for a foot that exhibits excessive pronation biomechanics.

neutral shoe—A running shoe with deformable, cushioning material throughout the entire length of the shoe and no foot pronation control material. This type of shoe is designed for a foot that exhibits typical pronation biomechanics.

pelvic drop—How much the hip drops on the opposite side of the single-support leg. With each step during gait, there is time spent standing on one leg, which is called single support. During single support, the pelvis, opposite to the stance limb, drops slightly. Excessive pelvic drop is associated with excessive hip adduction and knee abduction on the opposite (contralateral) side of the body and can create increased shearing forces within the pelvis, hip, and low back.

pes cavus—Indicative of a high arch measure and synonymous to a rigid foot and reduced foot pronation biomechanics.

pes planus—Indicative of a low arch (flat foot) measure and synonymous to a flexible foot and excessive foot pronation biomechanics.

prolonged pronation—The amount of time it takes for the foot to reach maximum pronation, which should occur around 50% of stance. The foot needs to complete pronation, get the big toe on the ground, and then begin to supinate (lock up) in order to form a rigid lever. The locked or supinated foot position produces a rigid lever in preparation for toe-off and maintains overall joint alignment. If the foot stays pronated for too long a period of time, twisting forces at the ankle and knee joint can occur. If the foot pronates too quickly, an increase in the shock wave of force traveling from the foot upward occurs, resulting in increased stress to the body.

pronation—Pronation is a combination of ankle dorsiflexion, rearfoot eversion, and forefoot abduction and occurs during the first half of stance. Pronation is synonymous to the foot unlocking and is necessary to accommodate to uneven surfaces, dissipate impact forces, and allow the big toe to reach the ground. Excessive foot pronation can cause the lower leg to rotate too far inward, which may increase twisting forces at the ankle and knee. Reduced foot pronation means the foot does not unlock and does not reduce the shock wave of force traveling from the foot upward, resulting in increased stress to the body. Foot pronation is also linked to knee and hip inward collapse.

Q-angle—The angle subtended by the line connecting the anterior superior iliac spine and the midpoint of the patella and one connecting the midpoint of the patella and the tibial tubercle.

rearfoot valgus (eversion)—A frontal plane motion and a component of foot pronation in which the rearfoot collapses inward. Rearfoot valgus can also refer to a standing posture measure in which the rearfoot (calcaneus) is orientated inward with respect to the ground.

rearfoot varus (inversion)—A frontal plane motion and a component of foot supination in which the rearfoot collapses outward. Rearfoot varus can also refer to a standing posture measure in which the rearfoot (calcaneus) is orientated outward with respect to the ground.

sagittal plane motion—Movement that occurs parallel to the midline of the body. For example, when observing a runner from the side, ankle flexion and knee flexion occur along the sagittal plane.

sampling frequency—Refers to the number of frames of data collected every second and measured in Hertz; sometimes referred to as sampling rate.

sampling theorem—Any biological signal should be sampled at least twice the rate of the highest frequency inherent in the signal itself. For example, if the movement occurs at 30 Hz, then the collection frequency (number of frames of data recorded per second) should be at least 60 Hz.

semicurved last—The amount of curvature for the shoe as measured by the long axis of the forefoot compared to the long axis of the rearfoot. A semicurved last refers to a 3° to 5° angulation between the forefoot and rearfoot with a slight inward foot flare.

shank—The lower aspect of the leg composed of the tibia and fibula bones. The shank includes the superior aspect of the ankle joint (along with the talus bone) and the inferior aspect of the knee joint.

shutter speed—The amount of time the volume of light coming through the lens, determined by the aperture or f-stop value, is allowed to stay on the film or digital media in the camera. Shutter speed is denoted as the inverse of one second: 1/500 indicates that the shutter will stay open for 1/500 of a second or 0.002 seconds. The longer the shutter speed, the more time light has to enter the camera and to be recorded.

stability shoe—A running shoe with some amount of foot pronation control material, such as higher density foam or a nondeformable material, placed near the arch or midfoot region of the shoe. This type of shoe has a balance between cushioning material and pronation control material. It is designed for runners who do not excessively pronate but have some foot characteristics, in combination with their overall foot mechanics, that place increased pronatory and torsional forces on their foot and lower leg while running.

standing rearfoot (shank/(tibial) angle—The angle subtended by the line along the long axis of the calcaneus and the long axis of the shank.

straight last—The last is the amount of curvature for the shoe as measured by the long axis of the forefoot compared to the long axis of the rearfoot. A straight last refers to no angulation between the forefoot and rearfoot. A straight last is concomitant with a 0° foot flare measure.

stride rate—The number of strides (footstrike to footstrike) taken every minute. This number depends on running velocity and is dependent on leg length as well as hip extension. There is no ideal stride rate but significant side-to-side differences are a good indicator of an antalgic gait pattern.

subtalar joint—Composed of the talus and calcaneus bones of the foot. The subtalar joint is immediately inferior to the talocrural joint. Rearfoot inversion and eversion occur at this joint.

supination—Supination is a combination of ankle plantar flexion, rearfoot inversion, and forefoot adduction and occurs during the second half of stance. Supination is synonymous to the foot locking and is necessary to create a rigid lever in order to propel the body forward and maintain forward running velocity. Excessive foot supination (synonymous to reduced foot pronation) can limit lower leg rotation, which may increase twisting forces at the ankle and knee. Supination means the foot remains locked and thereby does not reduce the shock wave of force traveling from the foot upward, resulting in increased stress to the body.

talocrural joint—Synonymous to the ankle joint and is composed of the tibia and fibula (bones of the shank) and the talus bone of the foot. Ankle plantar flexion and dorsiflexion occur at this joint.

tibial rotation—The maximum amount the lower leg rotates inward. This motion is mechanically coupled with foot pronation as well as hip and knee internal rotation. Too much or too little internal rotation creates increased twisting forces to the ankle and knee.

toe-out angle—The amount the foot angles away from the midline (duck-footed or pigeon-toed). Typically, a runner stands with the foot turned outward due to anatomical alignment. When running, however, the foot needs to be pointed more straightforward to reduce loading at the knee joint. A reduced or increased foot progression angle is needed to compensate for atypical hip, knee, and tibial rotation and rotation velocity. Significant side-to-side differences are a good indicator of an antalgic gait pattern.

transverse plane motion—Movement that occurs about, or around, the long axis of the body or a segment. For example, when observing a runner from above, tibial rotation and knee rotation occur along the transverse plane.

Weber-Barstow maneuver—Part of a clinical exam and a method to clear the hips and place them in a neutral position. The patient flexes both knees and hips, places the feet on the table, bridges the hips upward, and returns the hips to the table. The examiner holds the feet of the patient and places the thumbs over the medial malleoli while providing slight traction to extend the legs into a supine position.

References

Almeida, S., D. Trone, et al. 1999. Gender differences in musculoskeletal injury rates: A function of symptom reporting. *Med Sci Sports Exerc* 31(12): 1807-1812.

Almosnino, S., T. Kajaks, et al. 2009. The free moment in walking and its change with foot rotation angle. *Sports Med Arthrosc Rehabil Ther Technol* 1(1): 19.

Anderson, F.C., and M.G. Pandy. 2003. Individual muscle contributions to support in normal walking. *Gait Posture* 17(2): 159-169.

Areblad, M., B. Nigg, et al. 1990. Three-dimensional measurement of rearfoot motion during running. *J Biomech* 23(9): 933-940.

Arnold, A.S., F.C. Anderson, et al. 2005. Muscular contributions to hip and knee extension during the single limb stance phase of normal gait: A framework for investigating the causes of crouch gait. *J Biomech* 38(11): 2181-2189.

Bailon-Plaza, A., and M.C. van der Meulen. 2003. Beneficial effects of moderate, early loading and adverse effects of delayed or excessive loading on bone healing. *J Biomech* 36(8): 1069-1077.

Baitch, S.P., R.L. Blake, et al. 1991. Biomechanical analysis of running with 25 degrees inverted orthotic devices. *J Am Podiatr Med Assoc* 81(12): 647-652.

Barrios, J., K. Crossley, et al. 2010. Gait retraining to reduce the knee adduction moment through real-time visual feedback of dynamic knee alignment. *J Biomech* 43(11): 2208-2213.

Bates, B.T., L.R. Osternig, et al. 1979. Foot orthotic devices to modify selected aspects of lower extremity mechanics. *Am J Sports Med* 7(6): 338-342.

Birnbaum, K., C.H. Siebert, et al. 2004. Anatomical and biomechanical investigations of the iliotibial tract. *Surg Radiol Anat* 26(6): 433-446.

Blair, S., H. Kohl, et al. 1987. Rates and risks for running and exercise injuries: Studies in three populations. *Res Q Exerc Sport* 58: 221-228.

Blake, R., and J. Denton. 1985. Functional foot orthoses for athletic injuries: A retrospective study. *J Am Podiatr Med Assoc* 75(7): 359-362.

Blake, R.L. 1986. Inverted functional orthosis. *J Am Podiatr Med Assoc* 76(5): 275-276.

Bolgla, L., T. Malone, et al. 2008. Hip strength and hip and knee kinematics during stair descent in females with and without patellofemoral pain syndrome. *J Orthop Sports Phys Ther* 38(1): 12-18.

Brody, L., and J. Thein. 1998. Nonoperative treatment for patellofemoral pain. *J Orthop Sports Phys Ther* 28(5): 336-344.

Brouwer, A., A. van Tol, et al. 2007. Association between valgus and varus alignment and the development and progression of radiographic osteoarthritis of the knee. *Arthritis & Rheumatism* 56(4): 1204-1211.

Brown, G.P., R. Donatelli, et al. 1995. The effect of two types of foot orthoses on rearfoot mechanics. *J Orthop Sports Phys Ther* 21(5): 258-267.

Buchanan, K., and I. Davis. 2005. The relationship between forefoot, midfoot, and rearfoot static alignment in pain-free individuals. *J Orthop Sports Phys Ther* 35(9): 559-566.

Buchbinder, M.R., N.J. Napora, et al. 1979. The relationship of abnormal pronation to chondromalacia of the patella in distance runners. *J Am Podiatr Med Assoc* 69(2): 159-162.

Burnside, I., H. Tobias, et al. 1982. Electromyographic feedback in the remobilization of stroke patients: A controlled trial. *Arch Phys Med Rehabil* 63(5): 217-222.

Butler, R.J., I.S. Davis, et al. 2006. Interaction of arch type and footwear on running mechanics. *Am J Sports Med* 34(12): 1998-2005.

Byl, T., J. Cole, et al. 2000. What determines the magnitude of the Q-angle? A preliminary study of selected skeletal and muscular measures. *J Sports Rehabil* 9(1): 26-34.

Caspersen, C., K. Powell, et al. 1984. The incidence of injuries and hazards in recreational and fitness runners. *Med Sci Sports Exerc* 16: 113-114.

Cheung R.T., M.Y. Wong, and G.Y. Ng. Effects of motion control footwear on running: a systematic review. J Sports Sci. 2011 Sep;29(12):1311-9.

Cheung, R., and G. Ng. 2010. Motion control shoe delays fatigue of shank muscles in runners with overpronating feet. *Am J Sport Med* 38(3): 486-491.

Chumanov, E., B. Heiderscheit, et al. 2011. Hamstring musculotendon dynamics during stance and swing phases of high-speed running. *Med Sci Sports Exerc* 43(3): 525-532.

Cibulka, M., and J. Threlkeld-Watkins. 2005. Patellofemoral pain and asymmetrical hip rotation. *Phys Ther* 85(11): 1201-1207.

Cichanowski, H., J. Schmitt, et al. 2007. Hip strength in collegiate female athletes with patellofemoral pain. *Med Sci Sports Exerc* 39(8): 1227-1232.

Clarke, T., E. Frederick, et al. 1983. The effects of shoe design parameters on rearfoot control in running. *Med Sci Sports Exerc* 15(5): 376-381.

Clement, D.B., and J. Taunton. 1981. A guide to the prevention of running injuries. *Aust Fam Physician* 10(3): 156-161, 163-154.

Clement, D., J. Taunton, et al. 1981. A survey of overuse running injuries. *Physician Sports Med* 9(5): 47-58.

Colborne, G., S. Olney, et al. 1993. Feedback of ankle joint angle and soleus electromyography in the rehabilitation of hemiplegic gait. *Arch Phys Med Rehabil* 74(10): 1100-1106.

Colborne, G., F. Wright, et al. 1994. Feedback of triceps surae EMG in gait of children with cerebral palsy: A controlled study. *Arch Phys Med Rehabil* 75(1): 40-45.

Corkery, M., H. Briscoe, et al. 2007. Establishing normal values for lower extremity muscle length in college-age students. *Phys Ther Sport* 8(2): 66-74.

Cormack, S., K. Kendall, et al. 2011. Validation of 2D Measures of Hip and Knee Frontal Plane Biomechanics During Running. *J Athl Train* 46(3): s163.

Cornwall, M.W., and T.G. McPoil. 2004. Influence of rearfoot postural alignment on rearfoot motion during walking. *The Foot* 14(3): 133-138.

Cowan, D.N., B.H. Jones, et al. 1996. Lower limb morphology and risk of overuse injury among male infantry trainees. *Med Sci Sports Exerc* 28(8): 945-952.

Crenshaw, S.J., F.E. Pollo, et al. 2000. Effects of lateral-wedged insoles on kinetics at the knee. *Clin Orthop Relat Res* (375): 185-192.

Crowell, H., and I. Davis. 2011. Gait retraining to reduce lower extremity loading in runners. *Clin Biomech (Bristol, Avon)* 26(1): 78-83.

De Wit, B., and D. De Clercq. 2000. Timing of lower extremity motions during barefoot and shod running at three velocities. *J Appl Biomech* 16(2): 169-179.

De Wit, B., D. De Clercq, et al. 2000. Biomechanical analysis of the stance phase during barefoot and shod running. *J Biomech* 33(3): 269-278.

De Wit, B., D. De Clercq, et al. 1995. The effect of varying midsole hardness on impact forces and foot motion during foot contact in running. *J Appl Biomech* 11(4): 395-406.

DeHaven, K.E., and D.M. Lintner. 1986. Athletic injuries: Comparison by age, sport, and gender. *Am J Sports Med* 14(3): 218-224.

Derrick, T., G. Caldwell, et al. 2000. Modeling the stiffness characteristics of the human body while running with various stride lengths. *J Appl Biomech* 16(1): 36-51.

Dierks, T., and I. Davis. 2007. Discrete and continuous joint coupling relationships in uninjured recreational runners. *Clin Biomech (Bristol, Avon)* 22(5): 581-591.

Dierks, T., K. Manal, et al. 2008. Proximal and distal influences on hip and knee kinematics in runners with patellofemoral pain during a prolonged run. *J Orthop Sport Phys Ther* 38(8): 448-456.

Donatelli, R.A., C. Hurlburt, et al. 1988. Biomechanical foot orthotics: A retrospective study. *J Orthop Sport Phys Ther* 10(6): 205-212.

Donatelli, R., M. Wooden, et al. 1999. Relationship between static and dynamic foot postures in professional baseball players. *J Orthop Sport Phys Ther* 29(6): 316-325.

Duffey, M.J., D.F. Martin, et al. 2000. Etiologic factors associated with anterior knee pain in distance runners. *Med Sci Sports Exerc* 32(11): 1825-1832.

Dugan, S.A., and K.P. Bhat. 2005. Biomechanics and analysis of running gait. *Phys Med Rehabil Clin N Am* 16(3): 603-621.

Dye, S. 2001. Patellofemoral pain current concepts: An overview. *Sports Med Arthrosc Rev* 9: 264-272.

Dye, S., H. Staubli, et al. 1999. The mosaic of pathophysiology causing patellofemoral pain: Therapeutic implications. *Operative Tech Sports Med* 7: 46-54.

Earl, J., and A. Hoch. 2011. A proximal strengthening program improves pain, function, and biomechanics in women with patellofemoral pain syndrome. *Am J Sports Med* 39(1):154-63.

Eggold, J. 1981. Orthotics in the prevention of runners' overuse injuries. *Physician Sports Med* 9: 125-131.

Elliott, B. 1990. Adolescent overuse sporting injuries: A biomechanical review. *Australian Sports Commission Program*. 23: 1-9.

Eng, J.J., and M.R. Pierrynowski. 1993. Evaluation of soft foot orthotics in the treatment of patellofemoral pain syndrome. *Phys Ther* 73(2): 62-68; discussion 68-70.

Ferber, R. 2007. The influence of custom foot orthoses on lower extremity running mechanics. *Int SportMed J* 8(3): 97-103.

Ferber, R. and B. Benson. 2011. Changes in multi-segment foot biomechanics with a heat-mouldable semi-custom foot orthotic device. *J Foot Ankle Res* 4(1): 18.

Ferber, R., L. Bolgla, et al. 2011. Variability of hip and knee joint biomechanics during running for patients with patellofemoral pain syndrome. *J Athl Train* 46(3): S28.

Ferber, R., I.M. Davis, et al. 2003. Gender differences in lower extremity mechanics during running. *Clin Biomech (Bristol, Avon)* 18(4): 350-357.

Ferber, R., I.M. Davis, et al. 2005. Effect of foot orthotics on rearfoot and tibia joint coupling patterns and variability. *J Biomech* 38(3): 477-483.

Ferber, R., K. Kendall, et al. 2011. Changes in knee biomechanics following a hip abductor strengthening protocol for runners with patellofemoral pain syndrome. *Journal of Athletic Training* 46(2): 142-149.

Ferber R., K.D. Kendall, and L. McElroy. 2010. Normative and critical criteria for iliotibial band and iliopsoas muscle flexibility. *J Athl Train.* 45(4):344-348.

Ferber, R., B. Noehren, et al. 2010. Competitive female runners with a history of iliotibial band syndrome demonstrate atypical hip and knee kinematics. *J Orthop Sports Phys Ther* 40(2): 52-58.

Ferber, R., L.R. Osternig, et al. 2002a. Gait mechanics in chronic ACL deficiency and subsequent repair. *Clin Biomech (Bristol, Avon)* 17(4): 274-285.

Ferber, R., L.R. Osternig, et al. 2002b. Reactive balance adjustments to unexpected perturbations during human walking. *Gait Posture* 16(3): 238-248.

Ferber, R, L.R. Osternig, et al. 2003. Gait perturbation response in chronic anterior cruciate ligament deficiency and repair. *Clin Biomech (Bristol, Avon)* 18(2): 132-141.

Ferber, R., and M. Pohl. 2011. Changes in joint coupling and variability during walking following tibialis posterior muscle fatigue. *J Foot Ankle Res* 4(6): 1-8.

Ferber, R., K. Sheerin, et al. 2009. Measurement error of rearfoot kinematics during running between a 100Hz and 30Hz camera. *Int SportMed J* 10(3): 152-162.

Fields, K., J. Sykes, et al. 2010. Prevention of running injuries. *Current Sports Medicine Reports* 9(3): 176-182.

Finestone, A., V. Novack, et al. 2004. A prospective study of the effect of foot orthoses composition and fabrication on comfort and the incidence of overuse injuries. *Foot Ankle Int* 25(7): 462-466.

Fredericson, M., C.L. Cookingham, et al. 2000. Hip abductor weakness in distance runners with iliotibial band syndrome. *Clin J Sport Med* 10(3): 169-175.

Fulkerson, J.P. 2002. Diagnosis and treatment of patients with patellofemoral pain. *Am J Sports Med* 30(3): 447-456.

Garbalosa, J., M. McClure, et al. 1994. The frontal plane relationship of the forefoot to the rearfoot in an asymptomatic population. *J Orthop Sports Phys Ther* 20(4): 200-206.

Goonetilleke, R.S. and A. Luximon. 1999. Foot Flare and Foot Axis. *Human factors: The Journal of the Human Factors and Ergonomics Society* 41: 596.

Gross, M.L., L.B. Davlin, et al. 1991. Effectiveness of orthotic shoe inserts in the long-distance runner. *Am J Sports Med* 19(4): 409-412.

Hamill, J., B. Bates, et al. 1982. Comparisons between selected ground reaction force parameters at different running speeds. *Med Sci Sports Exerc* 14(2): 143.

Hamill, J., R.E. van Emmerik, et al. 1999. A dynamical systems approach to lower extremity running injuries. *Clin Biomech (Bristol, Avon)* 14(5): 297-308.

Hardin, E., A. Van Den Bogert, et al. 2004. Kinematic adaptations during running: Effects of footwear, surface, and duration. *Med Sci Sports Exerc* 36(5), 838-844.

Hart, L., S. Walter, et al. 1989. The effect of stretching and warmup on the development of musculoskeletal injuries (MSI) in distance runners. *Med Sci Sports Exerc* 21(Suppl): s59.

Harvey, D. 1998. Assessment of the flexibility of elite athletes using the modified Thomas test. *Br J Sports Med* 32(1): 68-70.

Heiderscheit, B., J. Hamill, et al. 1999. Q-angle influences on the variability of lower extremity coordination during running. *Med Sci Sports Exerc* 31(9): 1313-1319.

Heiderscheit, B., J. Hamill, et al. 2000. Influence of Q-angle on lower-extremity running kinematics. *J Orthop Sports Phys Ther* 30(5): 271-278.

Herrington, L., and C. Nester. 2004. Q-angle undervalued? The relationship between Q-angle and medio-lateral position of the patella. *Clin Biomech (Bristol, Avon)* 19(10): 1070-1073.

Hogue, R., and S. McCandless. 1983. Genu recurvatum: Auditory biofeedback treatment for adult patients with stroke or head injuries. *Arch Phys Med Rehabil* 64(8): 368-370.

Holden, J., and P. Cavanagh. 1991. The free moment of ground reaction in distance running and its changes with pronation. *J Biomech* 24(10): 887-897.

Horton, M.G., and T.L. Hall. 1989. Quadriceps femoris muscle angle: Normal values and relationships with gender and selected skeletal measures. *Phys Ther* 69(11): 897-901.

Hreljac, A. 2004. Impact and overuse injuries in runners. *Med Sci Sports Exerc* 36(5): 845-849.

Hreljac, A., R.N. Marshall, et al. 2000. Evaluation of lower extremity overuse injury potential in runners. *Med Sci Sports Exerc* 32(9): 1635-1641.

Hudson, Z., and E. Darthuy. 2009. Iliotibial band tightness and patellofemoral pain syndrome: A case-control study. *Man Ther* 14(2): 147-151.

Hung, Y.J., and M.T. Gross. 1999. Effect of foot position on electromyographic activity of the vastus medialis oblique and vastus lateralis during lower-extremity weight-bearing activities. *J Orthop Sports Phys Ther* 29(2): 93-102; discussion 103-105.

Hunt, A., R. Smith, et al. 2001. Inter-segment foot motion and ground reaction forces over the stance phase of walking. *Clin Biomech* 16(7): 592-600.

Inman, V. 1976. *The Joints of the Ankle*. Baltimore: Williams and Wilkins.

Intiso, D., V. Santilli, et al. 1994. Rehabilitation of walking with electromyographic biofeedback in foot-drop after stroke. *Stroke* 25(6): 1189-1192.

Ireland, M., J. Willson, et al. 2003. Hip strength in females with and without patellofemoral pain. *J Orthop Sports Phys Ther* 33(11): 671-676.

Jacobs, S.J., and B.L. Berson. 1986. Injuries to runners: A study of entrants to a 10,000 meter race. *Am J Sports Med* 14(2): 151-155.

James, S. 1998. Running injuries of the knee. *AAOS Instr Course Lect* 47:407-417.

James, S.L., B.T. Bates, et al. 1978. Injuries to runners. *Am J Sports Med* 6(2): 40-50.

James, S., and D. Jones. 1990. Biomechanical aspects of distance running injuries. *Biomechanics of Distance Running*. ed. P. Cavanagh. Champaign, IL: Human Kinetics: 249-269.

Kannus, P., L. Josza, et al. 1997. The effects of training, immobilization and remobilization on musculoskeletal tissues. *Scand J Med Sci Sports* 7(2): 67-71.

Kendall, K., K. Sheerin, et al. 2008. Normative database of common anatomical measures related to running injuries. *J Athl Train* 43(123).

Kernozek, T.W., and N.L. Greer. Quadriceps angle and rearfoot motion: relationships in walking. Arch Phys Med Rehabil. 1993 Apr;74(4):407-10.

Kerrigan, D.C., J.R. Franz, et al. 2009. The effect of running shoes on lower extremity joint torques. *PM R* 1(12): 1058-1063.

Kerrigan, D., A. Xenopoulos-Oddsson, et al. 2003. Effect of a hip flexor-stretching program on gait in the elderly. *Arch Phys Med Rehabil* 84(1): 1-6.

Kersting, U.G., and G.P. Bruggemann. 2006. Midsole material-related force control during heel-toe running. *Res Sports Med* 14(1): 1-17.

Kibler, W.B. 1990. Clinical aspects of muscle injury. *Med Sci Sports Exerc* 22(4): 450-452.

Kilmartin, T.E., and W.A. Wallace. 1994. The scientific basis for the use of biomechanical foot orthoses in the treatment of lower limb sports injuries--a review of the literature. *Br J Sports Med* 28(3): 180-184.

Kitaoka, H., Z. Luo, et al. 1997. Effect of posterior tibial tendon on the arch of the foot during simulated weightbearing: Biomechanical analysis. *Foot Ankle Int* 18(1): 43-46.

Klingman, R.E., S.M. Liaos, et al. 1997. The effect of subtalar joint posting on patellar glide position in subjects with excessive rearfoot pronation. *J Orthop Sports Phys Ther* 25(3): 185-191.

Knapik, J.J., L.C. Brosch, et al. 2010. Effect on injuries of assigning shoes based on foot shape in air force basic training. *Am J Prev Med* 38(1 Suppl): S197-211.

Knapik, J.J., A. Spiess, et al. 2010. Systematic review of the parachute ankle brace: Injury risk reduction and cost effectiveness. *Am J Prev Med* 38(1 Suppl): S182-188.

Knapik, J.J., D.I. Swedler, et al. 2009. Injury reduction effectiveness of selecting running shoes based on plantar shape. *J Strength Cond Res* 23(3): 685-697.

Konsgaard, M., C. Nielsen, et al. 2011. Mechanical properties of the human Achilles tendon, in vivo. *Clin Biomech* 26(7):772-777.

Koplan, J.P., K.E. Powell, et al. 1982. An epidemiologic study of the benefits and risks of running. *JAMA* 248(23): 3118-3121.

Landorf, K.B., and A.M. Keenan. 2000. Efficacy of foot orthoses. What does the literature tell us? *J Am Podiatr Med Assoc* 90(3): 149-158.

Leardini, A., M. Benedetti, et al. 2007. Rear-foot, mid-foot and fore-foot motion during the stance phase of gait. *Gait Posture* 25(3): 453-462.

Li, G., T.W. Rudy, et al. 1999. The importance of quadriceps and hamstring muscle loading on knee kinematics and in-situ forces in the ACL. *J Biomech* 32(4): 395-400.

Lieberman, D.E., M. Venkadesan, et al. 2010. Foot strike patterns and collision forces in habitually barefoot versus shod runners. *Nature* 463(7280): 531-535.

Livingston, L.A. 1998. The quadriceps angle: A review of the literature. *J Orthop Sports Phys Ther* 28(2): 105-109.

Livingston, L., and J. Mandigo. 1997. Bilateral within-subject Q angle asymmetry in young adult females and males. *Biomed Sci Instrum* 33:112-117.

Lundberg, A., O.K. Svensson, et al. 1989. Kinematics of the ankle/foot complex—part 3: Influence of leg rotation. *Foot Ankle* 9(6): 304-309.

Lysholm, J., and J. Wiklander. 1987. Injuries in runners. *Am J Sports Med* 15(2): 168-171.

Macera, C.A., S.A. Ham, et al. 2005. Prevalence of physical activity in the United States: Behavioral Risk Factor Surveillance System, 2001. *Prev Chronic Dis* 2(2): A17.

Macera, C.A., R.R. Pate, et al. 1989. Predicting lower-extremity injuries among habitual runners. *Arch Intern Med* 149(11): 2565-2568.

Macintyre, J., J. Taunton, et al. 1991. Running injuries: A clinical study of 4,173 cases. *Clin J Sports Med*: 1:81-87.

MacLean, C., I.M. Davis, et al. 2006. Influence of a custom foot orthotic intervention on lower extremity dynamics in healthy runners. *Clin Biomech (Bristol, Avon)* 21(6): 623-630.

Manter, J. 1941. Movements of the subtalar and transverse tarsal joints. *Anat Rec* 80: 397-410.

Marti, B., J. Vader, et al. 1988. On the epidemiology of running injuries: The 1984 Bern Grand-Prix study. *Am J Sports Med* 16(3): 285-293.

Mascal, C., R. Landel, et al. 2003. Management of patellofemoral pain targeting hip, pelvis, and trunk muscle function: 2 case reports. *J Orthop Sports Phys Ther* 33(11): 647-660.

Matheson, G.O., J.G. Macintyre, et al. 1989. Musculoskeletal injuries associated with physical activity in older adults. *Med Sci Sports Exerc* 21(4): 379-385.

McClay, I., and K. Manal. 1997. A comparison of three-dimensional lower extremity kinematics during running between excessive pronators and normals. *Clin Biomech* 13(3): 195-203.

McClay, I., and K. Manal. 1998. The influence of foot abduction on differences between two-dimensional and three-dimensional rearfoot motion. *Foot Ankle Int* 19(1): 26-31.

McClay, I., and K. Manal. 1999. Three-dimensional kinetic analysis of running: Significance of secondary planes of motion. *Med Sci Sports Exerc* 31(11): 1629-1637.

McClay, I., D. Williams, et al. 1999. Can Gait be Retrained to Prevent Injury in Runners? *American Society of Biomechanics*. Pittsburgh, PA.

McCulloch, M.U., D. Brunt, et al. 1993. The effect of foot orthotics and gait velocity on lower limb kinematics and temporal events of stance. *J Orthop Sports Phys Ther* 17(1): 2-10.

McGee, D. 2007. *Orthopedic Physical Assessment, 5th Ed.* . Philadelphia: W.B. Saunders Company.

McKenzie, D.C., D.B. Clement, et al. 1985. Running shoes, orthotics, and injuries. *Sports Med* 2(5): 334-347.

McLean, S., A. Su, et al. 2003. Development and validation of a 3-D model to predict knee joint loading during dynamic movement. *J Biomech Eng* 125(6): 864-874.

McPoil, T., B. Vicenzino, et al. 2009. Reliability and normative values for the foot mobility magnitude: A composite measure of vertical and medial-lateral mobility of the midfoot. *J Foot Ankle Res* 2:6.

McPoil, T.G., and M.W. Cornwall 2000. The effect of foot orthoses on transverse tibial rotation during walking. *J Am Podiatr Med Assoc* 90(1): 2-11.

McPoil, T.G., M.W. Cornwall, et al. 2008. Arch height change during sit-to-stand: an alternative for the navicular drop test. *J Foot Ankle Res* 1(1): 3.

Mercer, J.A., J. Vance, et al. 2002. Relationship between shock attenuation and stride length during running at different velocities. *Eur J Appl Physiol* 87(4-5): 403-408.

Messier, S.P., S.E. Davis, et al. 1991. Etiologic factors associated with patellofemoral pain in runners. *Med Sci Sports Exerc* 23(9): 1008-1015.

Messier, S.P., D.G. Edwards, et al. 1995. Etiology of iliotibial band friction syndrome in distance runners. *Med Sci Sports Exerc* 27(7): 951-960.

Messier, S.P., and K.A. Pittala. 1988. Etiologic factors associated with selected running injuries. *Med Sci Sports Exerc* 20(5): 501-505.

Milgrom, C., M. Giladi, et al. 1985. A prospective study of the effect of a shock-absorbing orthotic device on the incidence of stress fractures in military recruits. *Foot Ankle* 6(2): 101-104.

Miller, R.H., J.L. Lowry, et al. 2007. Lower extremity mechanics of iliotibial band syndrome during an exhaustive run. *Gait Posture* 26(3): 407-413.

Mills, K., P. Blanch, et al. 2010. Foot orthoses and gait: A systematic review and meta-analysis of literature pertaining to potential mechanisms. *Br J Sports Med* 44(14): 1035-1046.

Milner, C., I. Davis, et al. 2004. Is free moment related to tibial stress fracture in distance runners? *Med Sci Sports Exerc* 36: s57.

Milner, C., I. Davis, et al. 2006. Free moment as a predictor of tibial stress fracture in distance runners. *J Biomech* 39(15): 2819-2825.

Mizuno, Y., M. Kumagai, et al. 2001. Q-angle influences tibiofemoral and patellofemoral kinematics. *J Orthop Res* 19(5): 834-840.

Moore, K., and A. Dalley. 2005. *Clinically Oriented Anatomy*. Baltimore: Lippincott Williams & Wilkins.

Moraros, J., and W. Hodge. 1993. Orthotic survey: Preliminary results. *J Am Podiatr Med Assoc* 83(3): 139-148.

Morris, M., T. Matyas, et al. 1992. Electrogoniometric feedback: Its effect on genu recurvatum in stroke. *Arch Phys Med Rehabil* 73(12): 1147-1154.

Mundermann, A., B.M. Nigg, et al. 2003a. Foot orthotics affect lower extremity kinematics and kinetics during running. *Clin Biomech (Bristol, Avon)* 18(3): 254-262.

Mundermann, A., B.M. Nigg, et al. 2003b. Orthotic comfort is related to kinematics, kinetics, and EMG in recreational runners. *Med Sci Sports Exerc* 35(10): 1710-1719.

Mundermann, A., J.M. Wakeling, et al. 2006. Foot orthoses affect frequency components of muscle activity in the lower extremity. *Gait Posture* 23(3): 295-302.

Murley, G.S., H.B. Menz, et al. 2009. Foot posture influences the electromyographic activity of selected lower limb muscles during gait. *Journal of Foot and Ankle Research* 2: 35.

Naslund, J., S. Odenbring, et al. 2005. Diffusely increased bone scintigraphic uptake in patellofemoral pain syndrome. *Br J Sports Med* 39(3): 162-165.

Nawoczenski, D.A., T.M. Cook, et al. 1995. The effect of foot orthotics on three-dimensional kinematics of the leg and rearfoot during running. *J Orthop Sports Phys Ther* 21(6): 317-327.

Nawoczenski, D.A., and P.M. Ludewig. 1999. Electromyographic effects of foot orthotics on selected lower extremity muscles during running. *Arch Phys Med Rehabil* 80(5): 540-544.

Nawoczenski, D.A., C.L. Saltzman, et al. 1998. The effect of foot structure on the three-dimensional kinematic coupling behavior of the leg and rear foot. *Phys Ther* 78(4): 404-416.

Neptune, R.R., I.C. Wright, et al. 2000. The influence of orthotic devices and vastus medialis strength and timing on patellofemoral loads during running. *Clin Biomech (Bristol, Avon)* 15(8): 611-618.

Ness, M.E., J. Long, et al. 2008. Foot and ankle kinematics in patients with posterior tibial tendon dysfunction. *Gait Posture* 27(2): 331-339.

Nester, C.J., M.L. van der Linden, et al. 2003. Effect of foot orthoses on the kinematics and kinetics of normal walking gait. *Gait Posture* 17(2): 180-187.

Neufeld, S.K., and R. Cerrato. 2008. Plantar fasciitis: Evaluation and treatment. *J Am Acad Orthop Surg* 16(6): 338-346.

Niemuth, P.E., R.J. Johnson, et al. 2005. Hip muscle weakness and overuse injuries in recreational runners. *Clin J Sport Med* 15(1): 14-21.

Nigg, B. 1986. Biomechanical aspects of running. *Biomechanics of running shoes*. Champaign IL: Human Kinetics: 1-25.

Nigg, B.M., H.A. Bahlsen, et al. 1987. The influence of running velocity and midsole hardness on external impact forces in heel-toe running. *J Biomech* 20(10): 951-959.

Nigg, B.M., and M. Morlock. 1987. The influence of lateral heel flare of running shoes on pronation and impact forces. *Med Sci Sports Exerc* 19(3): 294-302.

Nigg, B.M., M.A. Nurse, et al. 1999. Shoe inserts and orthotics for sport and physical activities. *Med Sci Sports Exerc* 31(7 Suppl): S421-428.

Nigg, B.M., P. Stergiou, et al. 2003. Effect of shoe inserts on kinematics, center of pressure, and leg joint moments during running. *Med Sci Sports Exerc* 35(2): 314-319.

Noble, C.A. 1980. Iliotibial band friction syndrome in runners. *Am J Sports Med* 8(4): 232-234.

Noehren, B., I. Davis, et al. 2007. ASB clinical biomechanics award winner 2006 prospective study of the biomechanical factors associated with iliotibial band syndrome. *Clin Biomech (Bristol, Avon)* 22(9): 951-956.

Noehren, B., J. Scholz, et al. 2011. The effect of real-time gait retraining on hip kinematics, pain and function in subjects with patellofemoral pain syndrome. *Br J Sports Med* 45(9): 691-696.

Novick, A., and D.L. Kelley. 1990. Position and movement changes of the foot with orthotic intervention during the loading response of gait. *J Orthop Sports Phys Ther* 11(7): 301-312.

O'Connor, K., and J. Hamill. 2004. The role of selected extrinsic foot muscles during running. *Clin Biomech (Bristol, Avon)* 19(1): 71-77.

Olney, S., G. Colborne, et al. 1989. Joint angle feedback and biomechanical gait analysis in stroke patients: a case report. *Phys Ther* 69(10): 863-870.

Orchard, J.W., P.A. Fricker, et al. 1996. Biomechanics of iliotibial band friction syndrome in runners. *Am J Sports Med* 24(3): 375-379.

Osternig, L., R. Ferber, et al. 2000. Human hip and knee torque accommodations to anterior cruciate ligament dysfunction. *Euro J Appl Phys* 83(1): 71-76.

Pandy, M., and T. Andriacchi. 2010. Muscle and joint function in human locomotion. *Annu Rev Biomed Eng* 12: 401-433.

Pandy, M., Y. Lin, et al. 2010. Muscle coordination of mediolateral balance in normal walking. *J Biomech* 43(11): 2055-2064.

Pandy, M., and K. Shelburne. 1997. Dependence of cruciate-ligament loading on muscle forces and external load. *Journal of Biomechanics* 30(10): 1015-1024.

Paty, J.J. 1994. Running injuries. *Curr Opin Rheumatol* 6(2): 203-209.

Perttunen, J., E. Anttila, et al. 2004. Gait asymmetry in patients with limb length discrepancy. *Scand J Med Sci Sports* 14(1): 49-56.

Pinshaw, R., V. Atlas, et al. 1984. The nature and response to therapy of 196 consecutive injuries seen at a runners' clinic. *S Afr Med J* 65(8): 291-298.

Plastaras, C.T., J.D. Rittenberg, et al. 2005. Comprehensive functional evaluation of the injured runner. *Phys Med Rehabil Clin N Am* 16(3): 623-649.

Pohl, M.B., M. Rabbito, et al. 2010. The role of tibialis posterior fatigue on foot kinematics during walking. *J Foot Ankle Res* 3(6): 1-8.

Polk, J. 2005. Sampling frequencies and measurement error for linear and temporal gait parameters in primate locomotion. *J Hum Evol* 49(6): 665-679.

Powers, C. 1998. Rehabilitation of patellofemoral joint disorders: A critical review. 28(5): 345-354.

Powers, C. 2003. The influence of altered lower-extremity kinematics on patellofemoral joint dysfunction: a theoretical perspective. *J Orthop Sports Phys Ther* 33(11): 639-646.

Raissi, G., A. Cherati, et al. 2009. The relationship between lower extremity alignment and Medial Tibial Stress Syndrome among non-professional athletes. *Sports Med Arthrosc Rehabil Ther Technol* 1(1): 11.

Rattanaprasert, U., R. Smith, et al. 1999. Three-dimensional kinematics of the forefoot, rearfoot, and leg without the function of tibialis posterior in comparison with normals during stance phase of walking. *Clin Biomech (Bristol, Avon)* 14(1): 14-23.

Rauh, M., T. Koepsell, et al. 2007. Quadriceps angle and risk of injury among high school cross-country runners. *J Orthop Sports Phys Ther* 37(12): 725-733.

Richards, C., P. Magin, et al. 2009. Is your prescription of distance running shoes evidence based? *Br J Sports Med* 43(3): 159-162.

Robbins, S.E., and A.M. Hanna. 1987. Running-related injury prevention through barefoot adaptations. *Med Sci Sports Exerc* 19(2): 148-156.

Robinson, R., and R. Nee. 2007. Analysis of hip strength in females seeking physical therapy treatment for unilateral patellofemoral pain syndrome. *J Orthop Sports Phys Ther* 37(5): 232-238.

Rochcongar, P., J. Pernes, et al. 1995. Occurrence of running injuries: A survey among 1153 runners. *Science & Sports* 10: 15-19.

Rodgers, M.M., and B.F. Leveau. 1982. Effectiveness of foot orthotic devices used to modify pronation in runners. *J Orthop Sports Phys Ther* 4(2): 86-90.

Rolf, C. 1995. Overuse injuries of the lower extremity in runners. *Scand J Med Sci Sports* 5: 181-190.

Root, M., J. Weed, et al. 1966. Axis of motion of the subtalar joint. an anatomical study. *J Am. Podiatry Assoc* 56: 149-155.

Rose, H.M., S.J. Shultz, et al. 2002. Acute orthotic intervention does not affect muscular response times and activation patterns at the knee. *J Athl Train* 37(2): 133-140.

Rosenbloom, K.B. 2011. Pathology-designed custom molded foot orthoses. *Clin Podiatr Med Surg* 28(1): 171-187.

Ryan, M.B., G.A. Valiant, et al. 2011. The effect of three different levels of footwear stability on pain outcomes in women runners: a randomised control trial. *Br J Sports Med* 45(9): 715-721.

Saxena, A., and J. Haddad. 2003. The effect of foot orthoses on patellofemoral pain syndrome. *J Am Podiatr Med Assoc* 93(4): 264-271.

Seeger, B., D. Caudrey, et al. 1981. Biofeedback therapy to achieve symmetrical gait in hemiplegic cerebral palsied children. *Arch Phys Med Rehabil* 62(8): 364-368.

Seeger, B., and D. Caudrey. 1983. Biofeedback therapy to achieve symmetrical gait in children with hemiplegic cerebral palsy: Long-term efficacy. *Arch Phys Med Rehabil* 64(4): 160-162.

Silder, A., D. Thelen, et al. 2010. Effects of prior hamstring strain injury on strength, flexibility, and running mechanics. *Clin Biomech (Bristol, Avon)* 25(7): 681-686.

Smith, L.S., T.E. Clarke, et al. 1986. The effects of soft and semi-rigid orthoses upon rearfoot movement in running. *J Am Podiatr Med Assoc* 76(4): 227-233.

Snyder, K., J. Earl, et al. 2009. Resistance training is accompanied by increases in hip strength and changes in lower extremity biomechanics during running. *Clin Biomech* 24(1): 26-34.

Sobel, E., S. Levitz, et al. 1999. Natural history of the rearfoot angle: preliminary values in 150 children. *Foot Ankle Int* 20(2): 119-125.

Souza, R.B., and C.M. Powers. 2009. Differences in hip kinematics, muscle strength, and muscle activation between subjects with and without patellofemoral pain. *J Orthop Sports Phys Ther* 39(1): 12-19.

Stacoff, A., C. Reinschmidt, et al. 2000. Effects of foot orthoses on skeletal motion during running. *Clin Biomech (Bristol, Avon)* 15(1): 54-64.

Stanish, W.D. 1984. Overuse injuries in athletes: A perspective. *Med Sci Sports Exerc* 16(1): 1-7.

Stergiou, N., B.T. Bates, et al. 1999. Asynchrony between subtalar and knee joint function during running. *Med Sci Sports Exerc* 31(11): 1645-1655.

Subotnick, S. 1995. The biomechanics of running: Implications for the prevention of foot injuries. *Sports Med* 2(2): 144-153.

Swedler, D.I., J.J. Knapik, et al. 2010. Validity of plantar surface visual assessment as an estimate of foot arch height. *Med Sci Sports Exerc* 42(2): 375-380.

Taunton, J.E., M.B. Ryan, et al. 2002. A retrospective case-control analysis of 2002 running injuries. *Br J Sports Med* 36(2): 95-101.

Thijs, Y., D. Van Tiggelen, et al. 2007. A prospective study on gait-related intrinsic risk factors for patellofemoral pain. *Clin J Sport Med* 17(6): 437-445.

Thomee, R., J. Augustsson, et al. 1999. Patellofemoral pain syndrome: A review of current issues. *Sports Med* 28(4): 245-262.

Thordarson, D., H. Schmotzer, et al. 1995. Dynamic support of the human longitudinal arch: A biomechanical evaluation. *Clin Orthop Relat Res* 316: 165-172.

Tiberio, D. 1987. The effect of excessive subtalar joint pronation on patellofemoral mechanics: A theoretical model. *J Orthop Sports Phys Ther* 9(4): 160-165.

Tomaro, J., and R. Burdett. 1993. The effects of foot orthotics on the EMG activity of selected leg muscles during gait. *J Orthop Sports Phys Ther* 18(4): 532-536.

Tome, J., D. Nawoczenski, et al. 2006. Comparison of foot kinematics between subjects with posterior tibialis tendon dysfunction and healthy controls. *J Orthop Sports Phys Ther* 36(9): 635-644.

van der Worp, H., M. van Ark, et al. 2011. Risk factors for patellar tendinopathy: A systematic review of the literature. *Br J Sports Med* 45(5): 446-452.

van Mechelen, W. 1995. Can running injuries be effectively prevented? *Sports Med* 19(3): 161-165.

van Mechelen, W., H. Hlobil, et al. 1993. Prevention of running injuries by warm-up, cool-down, and stretching exercises. *Am J Sports Med* 21(5): 711-719.

Van Woensel, W., and P. Cavanaugh. 1992. A perturbation study of lower extremity motion during running. *Int J Sport Biomech* 8: 30-47.

Viitasalo, J.T., and M. Kvist. 1983. Some biomechanical aspects of the foot and ankle in athletes with and without shin splints. *Am J Sports Med* 11(3): 125-130.

Walter, S., L. Hart, et al. 1989. The Ontario Cohort Study of running-related injuries. *Arch Intern Med* 149: 2561-2564.

Wannstedt, G., and R. Herman. 1978. Use of augmented sensory feedback to achieve symmetrical standing. *Phys Ther* 58(5): 553-559.

Waryasz, G., and A. McDermott. 2008. Patellofemoral pain syndrome (PFPS): A systematic review of anatomy and potential risk factors. *Dyn Med.* 26: 7-9.

Watt, J., K. Jackson, et al. 2011. Effect of a supervised hip flexor stretching program on gait in frail elderly patients. *PM R* 3(4): 330-335.

Way, M.C. 1999. Effects of a thermoplastic foot orthosis on patellofemoral pain in a collegiate athlete: a single-subject design. *J Orthop Sports Phys Ther* 29(6): 331-338.

White S.C., L.A. Gilchrist, and B.E. Wilk. Asymmetric limb loading with true or simulated leg-length differences. Clin Orthop Relat Res. 2004 Apr;(421):287-92.

Willems, T.M., D. De Clercq, et al. 2006. A prospective study of gait related risk factors for exercise-related lower leg pain. *Gait Posture* 23(1): 91-98.

Willems, T., E. Witvrouw, et al. 2007. Gait-related risk factors for exercise-related lower-leg pain during shod running. *Med Sci Sports Exerc* 39(2): 330-339.

Williams, D., and I. McClay 2000. Measurements used to characterize the foot and the medial longitudinal arch: Reliability and validity. *Phys Ther* 80(9): 864-871.

Williams, D.I., I. McClay, et al. 2001. Arch structure and injury patterns in runners. *Clin Biomech (Bristol, Avon)* 16(4): 341-347.

Williams, D.S., 3rd, I. McClay Davis, et al. 2003. Effect of inverted orthoses on lower-extremity mechanics in runners. *Med Sci Sports Exerc* 35(12): 2060-2068.

Willson, J., and I. Davis. 2008. Utility of the frontal plane projection angle in females with patellofemoral pain. *J Orthop Sports Phys Ther* 38(10): 606-615.

Winter, D. 1982. Camera speeds for normal and pathological gait analyses. *Med Bio Eng Comp* 20(4): 408-412.

Winter, D. 1990. *Biomechanics and motor control of human movement.* New York: John Wiley and Sons.

Witvrouw, E., R. Lysens, et al. 2000. Intrinsic risk factors for the development of anterior knee pain in an athletic population: A two-year prospective study. *Am J Sports Med* 28(4): 480-489.

Witvrouw, E., S. Werner, et al. 2005. Clinical classification of patellofemoral pain syndrome: Guidelines for non-operative treatment. *Knee Surg Sports Traumatol Arthrosc* 13(2): 122-130.

Woodland, L.H., and R.S. Francis. 1992. Parameters and comparisons of the quadriceps angle of college-aged men and women in the supine and standing positions. *Am J Sports Med* 20(2): 208-211.

Yeung, E., and S. Yeung. 2001. A systematic review of interventions to prevent lower limb soft tissue running injuries. *Br J Sports Med* 35(6): 383-389.

Yoshioka, Y., D. W. Siu et al. 1989. Tibial anatomy and functional axes. *J Orthop Res.* 7(1): 132-137.

You, J., H. Lee, et al. 2009. Gastrocnemius tightness on joint angle and work of lower extremity during gait. *Clin Biomech* 24(9): 744-750.

Youdas, J., D. Krause, et al. 2005. The influence of gender and age on hamstring muscle length in healthy adults. *J Orthop Sports Phys Ther* 35(4): 246-252.

Index

Note: The italicized *f* and *t* following page numbers refer to figures and tables, respectively.

A
Achilles tendinitis 5*t*, 18, 32, 33
adductor magnus 47
adhesions 71
AHI. *See* arch height index
anatomical alignment. *See also* case studies; foot flare
  foot mechanics 18-20, 19*f*, 20*f*, 21*f*, 30-31, 31*f*, 44-45, 92-93
  hip mechanics 54-56, 55*f*, 96-97
  knee mechanics 44-46, 44*f*, 46*f*, 94-95
  tibial rotation 93
ankle motion
  flexibility factors 21, 56, 59
  footwear 26-27, 32, 34
  kinetic chain relationships 14, 38, 91-93, 107
  stance phase 11, 11*f*, 12*f*, 13*f*, 21, 38, 52
  strength factors 18, 67, 69, 71, 81
antalgic gait pattern 108, 109
anterior cruciate ligament 6, 42
aperture opening 102, 103
arch height index (AHI) 29-30, 30*f*, 67, 67*f*, 69, 71, 74, 80*f*, 92*t*, 93*t*
arch posture and motion. *See also* case studies
  biomechanics 12-13, 18, 19, 22
  footwear 23, 24-25, 27, 29-30, 30*f*, 34-35
  measuring arch height 29-30, 30*f*
  pes cavus 19, 24, 24*f*, 27, 30
  pes planus 19, 25, 27, 30
Areblad, M. 99
Arnold, A.S. 43
assessments, clinical and biomechanical
  biomechanical patterns
    foot, ankle, and tibia 91-93
    hip 91, 96-97, 98
    knee 91, 94-95, 98
case studies
  medial tibial stress syndrome 73-78, 74*f*, 75*f*, 76*f*, 77*f*, 84, 88-89
  patellofemoral pain syndrome 79-83, 80*f*, 81*f*, 82*f*, 84, 89

tibialis posterior tendinopathy 66-71, 67*f*, 68*f*, 70*f*, 84, 88-89

B
barefoot running 31-33
Barrios, J. 87
Bhat, K.P. 12
Bikila, Abebe 31-32
Bolga, L. 53
Buchanan, K. 20, 28-29
Budd, Zola 32
Butler, R.J. 30

C
calf muscles 18, 21, 32, 42, 66, 92, 93, 95
caliper measurements 30
camera systems vii, 99-103, 101*f*
cartilage breakdown 15, 41
case studies
  medial tibial stress syndrome 73-78, 74*f*, 75*f*, 76*f*, 77*f*, 84, 88-89
  patellofemoral pain syndrome 79-83, 80*f*, 81*f*, 82*f*, 84, 89
  tibialis posterior tendinopathy 66-71, 67*f*, 68*f*, 70*f*, 84, 88-89
Cavanagh, P. 56
center of mass 50, 52, 53, 53*f*
Chumanov, E. 47
Cibulka, M. 56-57
collection frequency 100-102, 101*f*
concentric phase 10, 10*f*, 11, 12*f*, 13*f*, 14-15, 19-20, 19*f*, 20*f*. *See also* stance phase
continuous relative phase (CRP) approach 44-45
core strength 88, 97
Corkery, M. 57-58
Cornwall, M.W. 12-13, 18, 20-21, 30
Crowell, H. 86-87
CRP. *See* continuous relative phase
cushioning phase 10, 10*f*, 11-14, 12*f*, 13*f*, 14*f*. *See also* stance phase

D

Dartfish 103
Darthuy, E. 59
Davis, I. 20, 28-29, 86-87
DgeeMe 103
Dierks, T. 53-54
digital cameras 100-102, 101*f*
distance considerations for training 2-3
Donatelli, R.A. 20, 33
dorsiflexion of the ankle 11, 11*f*, 12*f*, 21
Dugan, S.A. 12
Dye, S. 6

E

Earl, J. 88
eccentric phase 10, 10*f*, 11-14, 12*f*, 13*f*,
    14*f. See also* stance phase
electrogoniometers 86
electromyography (EMG) 86
eversion. *See also* pronation; rearfoot
    posture
    assessment tables for atypical action
        92-93
    biomechanics of the foot throughout
        stance 10*f*, 11, 11*f*, 12-14, 13*f*, 14*f*,
        38, 40, 93
    defining key terminology 107
    excessive peak rearfoot eversion
        anatomical alignment 18-20, 19*f*, 20*f*,
            22, 45, 67, 92
        biomechanics 92, 94, 95, 96, 108, 109
        definition 107
        flexibility factors 21, 72, 92
        injury assessment 59, 74, 76
        strength factors 16-18, 17*f*, 18-19,
            20-21, 22, 92
        video clips 15
    first ray mobility 20-21, 27
    footwear 24-25, 25*f*, 26-27, 26*f*, 33-34, 78
    free moment 56, 64, 65
    reduced peak rearfoot eversion
        anatomical alignment and flexibility
            20*f*, 74, 92
        biomechanics 92, 93, 94, 95, 96, 107
        video clips 16
    time to peak rearfoot eversion
        biomechanics 22, 92, 94, 96, 107, 109
        definition 107

injury assessment 15, 41, 74, 78, 81
velocity of rearfoot eversion 15, 74, 78,
    92, 93, 107
video analysis of rearfoot motion 99,
    100-102, 101*f*

F

feedback training 86-88. *See also* gait
    training
female runners and injury 6, 45-46, 47
femoral torsion 65, 98
Ferber, R. 101*f*
first ray mechanics 10, 12, 20-21, 22, 25,
    28, 56, 92
flare. *See* foot flare
flat feet 19, 25, 27, 30. *See also* arch pos-
    ture and motion
flexibility. *See also* case studies
    biomechani cs
        foot mechanics 20-21, 22, 64, 92-93
        hip mechanics 21, 56-61, 57*f*, 58*f*, 60*f*,
            96, 97
        knee mechanics 21, 47-48, 56-57, 95
        tibial rotation 93
    first ray mobility 20-21, 22, 25, 92
    gastrocnemius and soleus 18, 21, 42,
        66, 92, 93, 95
    hamstrings 47, 48
    iliotibial band 56, 57, 58, 59, 60*f*, 81, 83,
        95, 96
    quadriceps 47-48
    stretching 2, 3-4, 71
    Thomas tests 57-58, 57*f*, 58*f*
foot flare 24, 28-29, 28*f*
foot mechanics. *See also* case studies;
    eversion; pronation
    anatomical alignment 18-20, 19*f*, 20*f*,
        21*f*, 30-31, 31*f*, 44-45, 92-93
    arch deformation 12-13, 18, 19, 22,
        29-30, 30*f*
    assessment tables for atypical action
        92-93
    first ray mechanics 10, 12, 20-21, 22,
        25, 28, 56, 92
    flexibility factors 20-21, 22, 64, 92-93
    forefoot orientation 19-20, 19*f*, 20*f*, 21*f*,
        22, 24, 25, 28-29, 31*f*
    free moment 56, 64-65, 64*f*, 69

injuries
  Achilles tendinitis 5*t*, 18, 32, 33
  etiology 15-16, 18
  plantar fasciitis 5, 5*t*, 18, 34, 86
  kinetic chain relationships 91-93,
    94-95, 96-97, 107
  midfoot mobility 12-13
  plantar shapes 24, 28-29, 28*f*
  progression angles 64, 89, 96, 97, 98,
    109
  Q-angle 44-45, 44*f*
  rearfoot motion 10*f*, 11, 11*f*, 12-14, 13*f*,
    15-16, 18-19, 20-21, 93
  rearfoot orientation 18-19, 19*f*, 20, 20*f*,
    21*f*, 22
  stance phase mechanics 9-15, 10*f*, 11*f*,
    12*f*, 13*f*, 14*f*
  strength factors 16-19, 22, 64, 92-93
  video clips 12, 15, 16
foot strike. *See also* stance phase
  forefoot v. rearfoot striking pattern
    32-33
  gait biomechanics 10, 10*f*, 11-14, 12*f*,
    13*f*, 14*f*, 32-33, 109
  heel strike of the stance phase
    foot mechanics 11, 13*f*, 15
    hip mechanics 50, 50*f*, 51*f*, 52*f*
    injury etiology 16, 47, 61
    knee mechanics 42, 43*f*, 44
    muscle activity 41, 42, 43*f*, 44, 47
    shoes 24
    video analysis 100-102, 101*f*
footwear
  arch height index (AHI) 29-30, 30*f*
  barefoot running 31-33
  categories 24-25, 24*f*, 25*f*, 26*f*
  components 26-28, 28*f*
  last, shoe 24, 25, 25*f*, 28, 29
  orthotics 33-35
  prescription 22, 27-31, 28*f*, 29*f*, 30*f*, 31*f*
forefoot. *See also* stance phase
  neutral orientation 29
  shoe fitting 24, 28-29, 29*f*
  valgus orientation 19-20, 20*f*, 21*f*, 24,
    29
  varus orientation 19, 19*f*, 20, 21*f*, 22,
    25, 28-29, 31*f*
forefoot striking pattern 32-33

Francis, R.S. 45-46
Fredericson, M. 59, 61
free moment 56, 64-65, 64*f*, 69
frontal plane mechanics
  case study on medial tibial stress syn-
    drome 73-78, 74*f*, 75*f*, 76*f*, 77*f*, 84,
    88-89
  case study on patellofemoral pain syn-
    drome 79-83, 80*f*, 81*f*, 82*f*, 84, 89
  injury etiology 72
f-stop 102, 103

G
gait training 85-89
Garbalosa, J. 20
gastrocnemius muscle 21, 32, 42, 66,
  92, 93, 95
gender factors. *See* female runners and
  injury
genu valgum. *See also* medial tibial stress
  syndrome (MTSS); patellofemoral
  pain syndrome (PFPS)
  assessment tables 94
  definition 108
  foot mechanics 92, 93, 107
  gait training 86, 87
  hip mechanics 96, 108
  knee mechanics 38, 40*f*, 41, 94, 108
  muscular controls 53-54, 94
  pelvis mechanics 97, 108
  Q-angle 6, 44, 45, 94
  video clips 41
genu varum 40*f*, 92, 94, 96
gluteus muscles
  gait training 88-89
  hip mechanics 52-54, 52*f*, 61, 96
  injuries, gluteus medius 5*t*
  injury assessment 53-54, 61, 69, 71, 74,
    76, 78, 81, 83, 84
  knee mechanics 42, 44, 52-54, 94
  stride width 109
Goonetilleke, R.S. 25*f*, 28
Greer, N.L. 44

H
Haddad, J. 33
hamstring muscles
  flexibility 47, 48

hamstring muscles (*continued*)
  gait training 89
  hip mechanics 52-53, 52*f*
  injuries to the hamstrings 5*t*, 47
  knee mechanics 41-42, 42*f*, 43-44, 43*f*,
    94, 95
  strength assessment and injuries 69,
    71, 81, 83, 84
  tibia mechanics 93
Harvey, D. 48, 58
heel flare. *See* foot flare
heel strike
  foot mechanics 11, 13*f*, 15
  hip mechanics 50, 50*f*, 51*f*, 52*f*
  injury etiology 16, 47, 61
  knee mechanics 42, 43*f*, 44
  muscle activity 41, 42, 43*f*, 44, 47
  shoes 24
  video analysis 100-102, 101*f*
heel whip 64, 65, 65*f*, 69, 94, 96, 97
Heiderscheit, B. 45
Herrington, L. 46*f*
Hertz 100-102, 101*f*
high-speed cameras 100-102, 101*f*, 103
hip abductor muscles 7, 54, 61, 88, 94,
    96, 97
hip flexor muscles 59
hip mechanics. *See also* case studies
  anatomical alignment 54-56, 55*f*, 96-97
  assessment tables for atypical action
    96-97, 98
  barefoot running 32
  biomechanics across the kinetic chain
    92, 93, 94, 95, 107, 108
  feedback training 86, 87
  flexibility variables 21, 56-61, 57*f*, 58*f*,
    60*f*, 96, 97
  pronation factors 15
  Q-angle 96
  stance phase 50-52, 50*f*, 51*f*, 52*f*, 56
  strength factors 41, 52-54, 52*f*, 53*f*,
    56-57, 88
  terminology 108
  video clips 52, 53
  video gait analysis considerations 99
hip rotator muscles 41, 79, 81, 83, 86,
    93, 96, 97
Hoch, A. 88

Holden, J. 56
Hudson, Z. 59
Hunt, A. 13

I
iliopsoas 56, 57-59
iliotibial (IT) band
  anatomy and functions 59
  flexibility 56, 57, 58, 59, 60*f*, 81, 83, 95,
    96
  hip mechanics 96
  iliotibial band syndrome (ITBS) v, 5,
    5*t*, 6-7, 7*f*, 59, 61
  knee mechanics 43, 47, 59, 95
  tibia mechanics 93
individualization concepts 3-4
injuries. *See also* footwear
  overview of overuse injuries
    common running injuries v-vi, 4-7, 5*t*
    defining an overuse injury 1, 2
    etiology of overuse injuries 2-4, 2*f*, 5,
      7-8, 15-16
  risk factors
    assessment tables for atypical biome-
      chanics 91-98
    frontal plane forces 72
    leg length discrepancy 55
    Q-angle 6, 44-46, 44*f*, 46*f*, 74, 76
    stress-frequency relationship 2-3, 2*f*,
      4
    torsional forces 64-65
  stretching 2, 3-4, 71
  types
    Achilles tendinitis 5*t*, 18, 32, 33
    acute injuries 1
    iliotibial band syndrome v, 5, 5*t*, 6-7,
      7*f*, 59, 60*f*, 61
    medial tibial stress syndrome (MTSS)
      5*t*, 15, 73-78, 74*f*, 75*f*, 76*f*, 77*f*, 84,
      88-89
    muscle strains 1, 32, 47-48
    patellar tendinitis 5, 5*t*, 47-48
    patellofemoral pain syndrome (PFPS)
      case study 79-83, 80*f*, 81*f*, 82*f*, 84, 89
      etiology and biomechanical relation-
        ships 5-6, 15, 16, 41, 53-54, 57, 59
      feedback training 87
      orthotics 33

statistics of occurrence v, 5, 5*t*
strength training 83, 88
plantar fasciitis 5, 5*t*, 18, 34, 86
posterior tibialis tendon dysfunction (PTTD) 16-17, 17*f*
tibialis posterior tendinopathy 66-71, 67*f*, 68*f*, 70*f*, 84, 88-89
intensity considerations for training 2, 3
interrelationships. *See* assessments, clinical and biomechanical
inversion, rearfoot 10*f*, 11*f*, 13*f*, 14, 15, 16
IT. *See* iliotibial band
ITBSA. *See* iliotibial band syndrome

J
James, S.L. 33

K
Kendall, K. 30-31, 54, 55, 101*f*
Kernozek, T.W. 44
Kerrigan, D.C. 32, 58-59
kinetic-chain interrelationships. *See* assessments, clinical and biomechanical
knee mechanics. *See also* case studies
anatomical alignment 44-46, 44*f*, 46*f*, 94-95
assessment tables for atypical action 91, 94-95, 98
barefoot running 32
biomechanics across the kinetic chain 92, 93, 96, 97, 107, 108
feedback training 86, 87
flexibility factors 21, 47-48, 56-57, 59, 95
footwear 26-27, 33, 34
genu valgum 38, 40*f*, 41, 53-54, 94, 108
iliotibial band syndrome v, 5, 5*t*, 6-7, 7*f*, 59, 60*f*, 61
injury susceptibility v, 4, 5-6, 5*t*, 51-52
patellar displacement 45-46, 46*f*
patellar tendinitis 5, 5*t*, 47-48
patellofemoral pain syndrome
case study 79-83, 80*f*, 81*f*, 82*f*, 84, 89
etiology and biomechanical relationships 5-6, 15, 16, 41, 53-54, 57, 59
feedback training 87

orthotics 33
statistics of occurrence v, 5, 5*t*
strength training 83, 88
pronation impacts 14-15, 14*f*
stance phase 38-44, 38*f*, 39*f*, 40*f*, 51-52
strength factors 41-44, 42*f*, 43*f*, 56-57, 79
terminology 108
video clips 38, 41, 44, 48
video gait analysis 99
Kvist, M. 15

L
last, shoe 24, 25, 25*f*, 28, 29, 31, 31*f*
Leardini, A. 13
leg injuries 4, 5, 5*t*. *See also* shank mechanics
leg length discrepancy (LLD) 54-56, 55*f*
Li, G. 41-42
limb load monitors 86
limping gait pattern 108
Livingston, L.A. 45
LLD. *See* leg length discrepancy
lower leg. *See* shank mechanics
Lundberg, A. 40
Luximon, A. 25*f*

M
Manal, K. 99
Manter, J. 40
maps of biomechanical interrelationships. *See* tables assessing biomechanical patterns
Mar-Systems 103
McClay, I. 86, 99
McLean, S. 99, 103
McPoil, T.G. 12-13, 18, 20-21, 30
medial tibial stress syndrome (MTSS) 5*t*, 15, 73-78, 74*f*, 75*f*, 76*f*, 77*f*, 84, 88-89
meniscal injuries 5, 42
Messier, S.P. 61
midfoot mobility 12-13, 24, 25, 26*f*, 34
midsole hardness 26-27
Miller, R.H. 59-60
Mills, K. 33-34
Milner, C, 64
motion control running shoes 25, 25*f*, 26*f*, 27-28, 29, 30, 31, 31*f*, 74

MTSS. *See* medial tibial stress syndrome
muscles. *See* flexibility; strength training

N
navicular drop test 29
Nester, C. 46*f*
neutral running shoes 24, 24*f*, 25*f*, 29,
    30, 31, 31*f*, 71, 83
Noehren, B. 61, 87

O
Ober's Test 58, 59, 60*f*
Orchard, J.W. 6
orthotics 33-35, 71
osteoarthritis 87

P
Pandy, M. 41-42, 53
patellar displacement 45-46, 46*f*
patellar tendinitis 5, 5*t*, 47-48
patellofemoral pain syndrome (PFPS)
  case study 79-83, 80*f*, 81*f*, 82*f*, 84, 89
  etiology and biomechanical relation-
    ships 5-6, 15, 16, 41, 53-54, 57, 59
  feedback training 87
  orthotics 33
  statistics of occurrence v, 5, 5*t*
  strength training 83, 88
pelvis. *See also* case studies
  alignment measures 54
  atypical drop and stress 7*f*, 53, 94, 96,
    97, 108
  biomechanics 50, 56, 108
Perttunen, J. 56
pes cavus 19, 24, 24*f*, 27, 30. *See also*
    tibialis posterior muscles
pes planus 19, 25, 27, 30
PFPS. *See* patellofemoral pain syndrome
plane mechanics, frontal
  case study of medial tibial stress syn-
    drome 73-78, 74*f*, 75*f*, 76*f*, 77*f*, 84,
    88-89
  case study of patellofemoral pain syn-
    drome 79-83, 80*f*, 81*f*, 82*f*, 84, 89
  injury etiology 72
plantar fasciitis 5, 5*t*, 18, 34, 86
plantar flexion 10*f*, 11, 12*f*
plantar shapes 24, 28-29, 28*f*

popliteus 43
posterior tibialis tendon dysfunction
    (PTTD) 16-17, 17*f*
Powers, C.M. 57
progression considerations for training
    2, 3
pronation. *See also* eversion
  anatomical alignment 18-19, 19*f*, 20*f*
  flexibility factors 20-21
  footwear 23, 24-25, 27, 29
  free moment 56, 64-65, 64*f*
  knee mechanics 94
  prolonged pronation 14-15, 16, 22
  stance phase mechanics 10-12, 10*f*, 11*f*,
    14-15, 38, 107
  strength factors 16-19
  tibia mechanics 93
propulsion phase 10, 10*f*, 11, 12*f*, 13*f*,
    14-15, 19-20, 19*f*, 20*f*. *See also* stance
    phase
PTTD. *See* posterior tibialis tendon dys-
    function

Q
Q-angle
  assessment tables for atypical biome-
    chanics 94, 96
  gender comparison 45-46
  injury mechanics 6, 44-46, 44*f*, 46*f*, 74,
    76
  measuring 44*f*, 45-46
quadriceps muscle
  flexibility 47-48
  strength 41-42, 42*f*, 43, 43*f*, 44

R
Rauh, M. 46
rearfoot posture. *See also* eversion
  Q-angle impacts 44-45
  rearfoot-shank angles 30-31, 31*f*
  valgus orientation 18-19, 19*f*, 31, 31*f*
  varus orientation 20, 20*f*, 31, 31*f*
rearfoot striking pattern. *See* heel strike
rectus femoris 42, 56, 57-58, 81, 83
Richards, C. 23, 28
road maps to biomechanical interrela-
    tionships. *See* tables assessing bio-
    mechanical patterns

Root, M. 40
Running Injury Clinic vii, 8, 98
Ryan, M.B. 5*t*, 23

S
sampling frequency 100-102, 101*f*, 102
sampling theorem 100
sartorius 42-43, 47
Saxena, A. 33
scar tissue 47, 71
shank mechanics. *See also* orthotics
 assessment tables for atypical biomechanics 92, 93
 biomechanics across the kinetic chain
  92, 93, 94, 95, 96, 97, 98, 107, 108,
  109
 injuries
  medial tibial stress syndrome 5*t*, 15,
   73-78, 74*f*, 75*f*, 76*f*, 77*f*, 84, 88-89
  stress fractures 5*t*, 64, 87
 Q-angle impacts 44-45
 real-time feedback and alterations
  86-87
 rearfoot-shank angles 30-31, 31*f*
 stance phase 10*f*, 11, 13-15, 13*f*, 14*f*,
  50-51, 65
 terminology 107
Sheerin, K. 101*f*
Shelburne, K. 41-42
shin splints 5*t*, 15, 73-78, 74*f*, 75*f*, 76*f*,
  77*f*, 84, 88-89
shoes. *See* footwear
shutter speed 102, 103
Silder, A. 47
Silicon Coach 103
Snyder, K. 54, 88
Sobel, E. 30
software for 2D video analysis 103
soleus muscle 18, 21, 32, 42, 66, 92,
  93, 95
Souza, R.B. 57
speed considerations for training 2, 3
Sports Motion 103
stability running shoes 24-25, 25*f*, 26*f*,
  28, 29, 30, 31, 31*f*, 71, 78
stance phase. *See also* torsional forces
 anatomical alignment relationships
  19-20, 19*f*, 20*f*

foot mechanics 9-15, 10*f*, 11*f*, 12*f*, 13*f*,
  14*f*
 heel whip 64, 65, 65*f*
 knee mechanics 38-41, 38*f*, 39*f*, 40*f*, 48
 muscle activity 16-19, 17*f*, 41-44, 42*f*,
  43*f*, 47
 terminology 107-109
 video gait analysis 100-102, 101*f*
strength relationships. *See also* case
  studies
 foot mechanics 16-19, 22, 64, 92-93
 hip mechanics 41, 52-54, 52*f*, 53*f*, 56-57,
  96, 97
 knee mechanics 41-44, 42*f*, 43*f*, 94, 95
 tibial rotation 93
strength training 71, 78, 83, 88-89
stress fractures v, 5*t*, 64, 87
stress-frequency relationship 2-3, 2*f*, 4.
  See also injuries
stretching 2, 3-4, 71. *See also* flexibility
stride rate and length 32, 41, 47, 58,
  59, 109
stride-to-stride knee joint variability
  54, 88
stride width 109
subtalar joint axis 40
supination
 shoe prescription 24, 24*f*, 29, 31, 31*f*
 stance phase 10, 10*f*, 11, 11*f*, 12, 14
swing phase 41, 42*f*, 47

T
tables assessing biomechanical patterns.
  See also case studies
 foot, ankle, and tibia 91-93
 hip 91, 96-97, 98
 knee 91, 94-95, 98
talus movement 14, 14*f*, 40, 65
tarsal tunnel syndrome 66
Taunton, J.E. 5*t*
tensor fasciae latae 43, 59
Thijs, Y. 16
Thomas tests 57-58, 57*f*, 58*f*
3D motion capture systems vii, 99-100,
  103
Threlkeld-Watkins, J. 56-57
Tiberio, D. 40, 41
tibialis anterior muscles 17

tibialis posterior muscles
foot mechanics 16-19, 17*f*, 22, 92, 93
medial tibial stress syndrome 74, 76, 78
tibial internal rotation 93
tibialis posterior tendinopathy (TPT) 66-71, 67*f*, 68*f*, 70*f*, 84, 88-89
tibia mechanics. *See also* orthotics
assessment tables for atypical internal rotation 92, 93
biomechanics across the kinetic chain 92, 93, 94, 95, 96, 97, 98, 107, 108, 109
injuries
medial tibial stress syndrome 5*t*, 15, 73-78, 74*f*, 75*f*, 76*f*, 77*f*, 84, 88-89
stress fractures 5*t*, 64, 87
Q-angle impacts 44-45
real-time feedback and alterations 86-87
rearfoot-shank angles 30-31, 31*f*
stance phase 10*f*, 11, 13-15, 13*f*, 14*f*, 38-41, 50-51, 65
terminology 107
toe-off. *See also* stance phase
foot mechanics 10, 10*f*, 11, 12*f*, 13*f*, 14-15, 19-20, 19*f*, 20*f*
free moment 56, 64-65, 64*f*, 69
hip mechanics 50, 50*f*, 51*f*, 52*f*
muscle activity 41, 42*f*
toe-out angle 89, 96, 97, 98
torsional forces
case study on tibialis posterior tendinopathy 64-71, 64*f*, 65*f*, 67*f*, 68*f*, 70*f*
free moment 56, 64-65, 64*f*, 69
shoes 25
strength and flexibility factors 18, 56, 57, 61, 64
training variables 3
TPT. *See* tibialis posterior tendinopathy
training variables and injury risks 2-4, 2*f*, 71

truncated foot length 29, 30*f*
2D camera systems 99-103, 101*f*

V
valgus angles. *See* anatomical alignment; case studies
van der Worp, H. 47-48
varus angles. *See* anatomical alignment; case studies
vasti muscles 42, 43, 48, 52, 53, 81, 83, 95
Vicon Motus 103
video clips
case study on medial tibial stress syndrome 73
case study on patellofemoral pain syndrome 79
foot mechanics 12, 15, 16
heel whip 65*f*
hip mechanics 52, 53
knee mechanics 38, 41, 44, 48
tibialis posterior tendinopathy 66
using the online video vi, ix-x
video gait analysis vii, 99-103, 101*f*
Viitasalo, J.T. 15

W
Watt, J. 59
Weber-Barstow maneuver 54, 55*f*
wet test 28, 28*f*
White, S.C. 56
Willems, T.M. 15-16
Williams, D.S., III 34
Woodland, L.H. 45-46

Y
Yeung, E. 3-4
Yeung, S. 3-4
Yoshioka, Y. 6
Youdas, J. 47

About the Authors

Reed Ferber, PhD, CAT(C), ATC, is an associate professor in the faculties of kinesiology and nursing at the University of Calgary and cofounder and director of the Running Injury Clinic in Calgary, Alberta, Canada. Since 2003, he and his colleagues at the Running Injury Clinic have been among the world's leaders in 3-D gait assessment and technology. Ferber received his PhD in biomechanics from the University of Oregon in 2001. He is a research associate for the Institute of Sport and Recreation Research in New Zealand and a certified member of the Canadian Athletic Therapists' Association and the National Athletic Trainers' Association. He has won several awards in teaching excellence and has 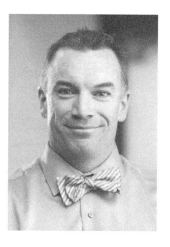 authored or coauthored 43 articles appearing in *Clinical Biomechanics, Gait and Posture, Clinical Journal of Sports Medicine, Journal of Sport Rehabilitation,* and other publications.

Shari Macdonald, MSc, BScPT, has worked for over 15 years as a physical therapist specializing in the assessment and treatment of musculoskeletal injuries. She has earned postgraduate certifications in manual therapy, dry needling techniques, and sport. Shari is the chairperson for the Alberta section of Sport Physiotherapy Canada and is a national board member. Since 2009, Shari has been the clinic director at the Running Injury Clinic in Calgary, Alberta, where they specialize in assessing gait biomechanics and the treatment of running injuries. Shari earned her master of science degree in biomechanics from the University of Calgary.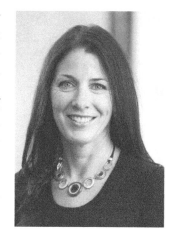

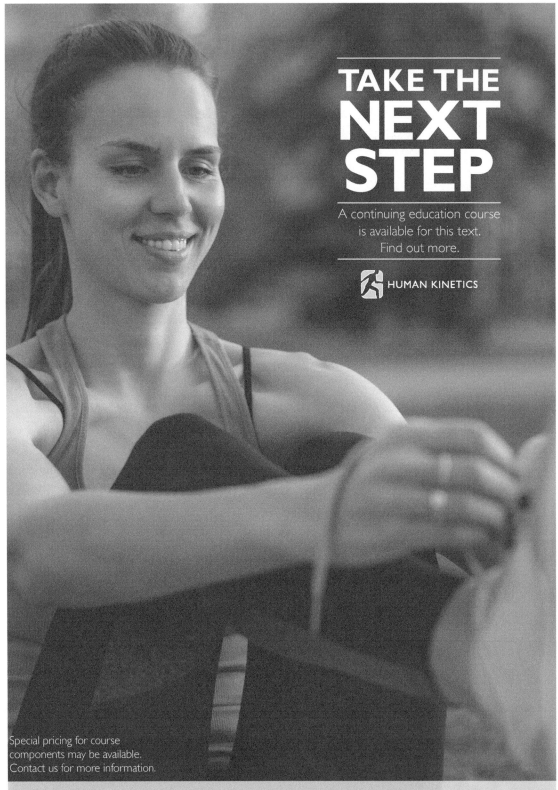